CANNABIS for Chronic Medical Conditions

The Path to be Well

Doug Rawson • Mark Tremblay • Paul Caluori

Cannabis for Chronic Medical Conditions

tellwell

Tellwell Talent
www.tellwell.ca

ISBN
978-0-2288-4091-6 (Hardcover)
978-0-2288-4090-9 (Paperback)
978-0-2288-4092-3 (eBook)

Table of Contents

Disclaimer

This book is intended for individuals who are generally well-adjusted, functioning effectively, and have overall good health, e.g. those who are not in need of medical treatment (including for mental health disorders). This book and its resources do not provide diagnoses for any medical or mental disorders, neither does this book prevent, cure, or treat any mental disorder or medical disease. Furthermore, this book and its resources are not a substitute for therapy, counselling, psychoanalysis, medical treatment, substance abuse treatment, or the advice or services of a medical professional. It is your responsibility to seek independent guidance from medical professionals to the extent necessary.

Dedication

To my family:
Charity, Anthony and Nikolas.
Thank you for your love and support.

—Paul Caluori

To family members who have inspired me on this journey—

My stepson Justin who introduced me to the notion of cannabis as a medicine and provided me an opportunity to help those that would benefit from cannabis therapy. My dear wife, who by stepping outside of her comfort zone, allowed me to witness firsthand how cannabis can help alleviate symptoms and improve sleep. My eighty-nine-year-old father who spent a lifetime helping those in need and inspired me to help those in my sphere of influence.

—Mark Tremblay

I have so many people to thank for their friendship, support, and love throughout my journey. To the many wonderful people, I have crossed paths with since beginning as a paramedic so many years ago. I have learned something from everyone and hope their teachings are relevant in this book. To my dad who is my biggest supporter, I appreciate all you offer and do, and for always being there. To my late mother, I cannot say how much I miss you, and how I wish I could share so much more with you. Most importantly, to my family, Dawn, Alex, Reid and Morgan. My love, focus and dedication to you is never-ending. Thank you. I am so proud of each of you, and I love all of you more than you will ever know. Thanks for your love and support and always being amazing!

—Doug Rawson

Foreword

If you are suffering from a medical condition and want to know if medical marijuana may be an effective treatment for you, then I encourage you to read this book.

The team at WeedWell™ is passionate about seeing people's lives change and be impacted in a positive way. I can state from a medical professional's point of view that the position this book takes with support and guidance is fair, responsible and safe. I cannot emphasize enough the importance of working with your health-care provider. The information, tips, tools and strategies discussed in this book follow a safe approach.

One of the most profound benefits of medicinal marijuana is its ability to reduce opiate use and soothe pain.

As a longtime emergency room physician, I can't think of anything more profound in the utilization of medicinal marijuana than that. Producing medical marijuana in accordance with government regulations can help to assure the quality and lack of contaminants and diluents. Like pharmaceutical medications, when the bottle says there's something specific inside it, I can be assured that what's on the label is what's in the bottle.

I am an actively practicing, board-certified emergency physician with over thirty years of experience working in the emergency department. I own and operate several urgent care facilities in central and south Florida. I am the Medical Director for several Fire Rescue and Emergency Medical Ambulance Services.

I know that life can be a struggle when you're living with a chronic disease or illness. This is because every day you realize that you have another whole day of pain or suffering ahead. You don't just want to feel better. You *need* to feel better. Medical marijuana may be right for you.

Getting information and support in creating a treatment plan that includes medical marijuana can be a frustrating and daunting task. After reading this book, use the strategies and work with your health-care provider in designing a treatment plan that works for you.

—J. M. Adelberg, MD, FAEP

Preface

Welcome and thank you for making an investment in your health with the purchase of this book.

This book would not be possible without the confidence entrusted in us by the thousands of clients we have had the privilege of serving.

Let us share our vision.

We are vigorously committed to our goal in helping 100,000 people who suffer from a chronic medical condition feel better by considering the safe use of cannabis in their treatment plan.

Chapter 1: Introduction

This book is written for people who want to gain confidence in using cannabis as part of their treatment. *Feeling better is possible.*

Oftentimes, we found that individuals suffering from a chronic medical condition were frustrated. They were wondering why finding a solution to their problem was so difficult. Many individuals have begun feeling better by completing some of the milestones discussed in this book.

Our focus is on getting you results. By gaining clarity on your health, you can establish your health goals aligned with your treatment plan. Celebrating small wins as you feel better will help you gain confidence in your treatment.

Your journey is divided into five stages, each building on the previous stage. The content of this book, *Cannabis for Chronic Medical Conditions: The Path to Be Well*, is based on our extensive clinical work, serving over 5,000 clients. This book is supported with over one hundred reputable sources. This book is not a 'pro cannabis' book. It is about supporting and guiding you on your health journey, while working in a safe and collaborative manner with your health-care team.

Don't settle for the status quo. If you are looking for a change, continue reading and start enjoying life with friends and family.

1.2 Introducing The Path to Be Well

The Path to Be Well is an outline of action items and milestones that we have designed to help you achieve your desired results. This first chapter is an introduction and overview of The Path to Be Well.

Chapter 2: Be Clear is the first stage of The Path to Wellness. Clients in this stage are frustrated with their chronic condition and believe that getting help is so difficult. This stage is focused on helping you gain clarity about your current state of health.

Chapter 3: Be Aware is the second stage of The Path to Wellness. Clients are often skeptical about the information available regarding medical cannabis and how it can relate to their individual needs. The milestone for this chapter is to set health goals that are important to you.

Chapter 4: Be Informed is the third stage of your wellness journey. Consumers are usually concerned about getting high. They have many questions about how to consume cannabis in a healthy way. The goal for this chapter is to understand cannabinoids and consumption methods while designing a treatment plan.

Chapter 5: Be Progressing is the fourth stage. Consumers hope they can find relief by accessing the right product. This chapter will discuss initiating and titrating your treatment plan while journaling for results.

This final stage is **Chapter 6: Be Well**. Consumers now take an active role in managing their healthcare. This chapter focuses on comparing and contrasting your health, providing clarity on your future Path to Wellness.

Chapter 2: Be Clear

Stage Characteristic

I am suffering from a chronic condition and frustrated that getting help is so difficult.

2.1 Your Health Selfie

Where Are You Starting on Your Journey?

Let's begin with where you are starting on your journey. Think of this as a selfie that you can look back on and use as a measuring stick to evaluate your success.

To create your selfie, you will need to gather information about your specific health conditions. This is a list of the conditions you are currently treating. Remember, your doctor can be an essential partner in your discovery.

Next, make a list of all the medications and supplements you are taking. While it is not necessary to understand how medicine works on a molecular level, it is vital that you understand the reasons for taking any medication. Take time to obtain clarity as to why you are being prescribed these medications. Your pharmacist can also help you understand the role of medication in your current treatment plan.

Please note: we are not suggesting that medications are not essential or required. In fact, many are needed and can be disease-altering, lifesaving, or symptom-relieving medications.

Expert Tip

Do not stop or change your medications without professional advice from your physician.

What is Positive and What is Limiting About Your Current State of Health?

The objective of this section is to get clear on your health. We want you to evaluate your mental, social, and physical well-being. Assess whether you have any factors affecting your mental, social, and physical well-being and consider ways to implement changes to improve your current state of health.

Some factors to consider when examining your physical well-being:

- Am I able to sleep?
- Do I wake up tired?
- Do I have pain?
- Does pain limit me?
- Are there things I want to do but can't anymore?
- Do I require mobility devices?

After evaluating and considering the factors affecting you, document strategies you can implement to improve your overall physical well-being.

Now, onto your mental well-being. Some questions to ask yourself:

- Am I in a good mental state right now?
- Do I feel like a burden on those around me?
- Do I feel like worthless?
- Is my depression out of control?
- Does my anxiety prevent me from doing things I want to do?

After evaluating and considering the factors affecting you, document strategies you can implement to improve your mental health.

Finally, let us look at social well-being. Look at the relationships around you and how they contribute to or hinder your life.

- Are my relationships healthy?
- Is my support system strong?
- Are my connections strong?
- Are my relationships suffering because of how I feel physically or mentally?
- Do I have family and friends whom I can confide in?

After evaluating and considering the factors affecting you, document strategies you can implement to improve your overall social well-being.

Helpful Resource

To access the Well-Being templates, visit: mypathtobewell.com.

You should be starting to get a more complete picture of yourself. This is an important foundational step that you will begin to build upon.

2.2 Be Clear About Your Mental Health

Let us begin by asking a question. If a friend or family member wanted to speak to you about their health issues, what would be the first thought to come to your mind?

Would you be wondering whether they are going to tell you they have a heart problem? Diabetes? Cancer? Or maybe that they are suffering from pain? Would it be fair to say that those first thoughts that come to your mind do not involve mental health? Why might that be?

Often, mental health is not something people talk about; perhaps due to stigma. Perhaps because there are no physical scars.

What is Mental Health?

The Public Health Agency of Canada defines positive mental health as "the capacity of each and all of us to feel, think and act in ways that enhance our ability to enjoy life and deal with the challenges we face" (PHAC, 2021). The Mental Health Commission of Canada stipulates that "mental health influences the way we think and feel about ourselves and others and how we interpret events. It affects our ability to learn, communicate and form, sustain or end relationships. It also influences our ability to cope with change." (Mental Health Commission of Canada, 2010).

Having a mental illness does not mean you cannot have good mental health. Having a solid understanding of your own state of mental health is fundamental to your journey.

How Clinicians Make a Diagnosis

Diagnosing mental health disorders can be a difficult process. It is challenging because many of the symptoms of mental health disorders can be the result of another condition. The *Diagnostic and Statistical Manual, 5th Edition* (or DSM-5) is a reference used by clinicians to diagnose mental disorders. The DSM-5 provides a standard for diagnosing mental health disorders. Mental health disorders are often diagnosed after eliminating other possibilities for the same symptoms (Depression Definition and DSM-5 Diagnostic Criteria, n.d.).

The scope of this book is not to provide a diagnosis for your mental health.

Expert Tip

If you are experiencing mental health symptoms, it is important to have a discussion with your primary care provider to get a professional assessment.

2.3 Be Clear About Your Pain

Pain is the most common condition treated with cannabis (Mastroianni, 2019). Traditional treatments and therapies may not provide you relief. Many are discouraged, even frustrated that getting help is so difficult. Some turn to cannabis as an alternative.

Before we begin to describe how cannabis may or may not be a viable treatment option, let us explore the types and classifications of pain.

What is Pain?

Let us start with how you experience pain. For example, back pain could be nerve related or due to tight muscles. Although the location of pain is in the back, it is experienced in your brain (Rath, 2021).

There are two main classifications of pain: time frame and source.

The Differences Between Acute and Chronic Pain

In general, pain classified by its time frame defines acute pain to be less than six months in duration, while chronic pain lasts longer than six months (Santos-Longhurst, 2018).

Classifying pain by source is the second method of classification. Pain, whether acute or chronic, can also be classified by its source. Classifying pain is important because treatments vary based on different types of pain.

Sources of Chronic Pain

Treede et al. describes the common types of chronic pain (2015):

- chronic cancer pain—due to cancer itself or cancer treatments
  eg. tumour or radiation burns
- chronic post-traumatic or post-surgical pain—pain that exists beyond the normal time for healing
  eg. car accident, trauma from a surgery itself
- chronic neuropathic pain—injury or dysfunction to the nervous system
- chronic visceral pain—pain that comes from the internal organs
  eg. Crohn's disease, ulcerative colitis
- chronic musculoskeletal pain—comes from a disease affecting the tissues of muscles and joints
  eg. rheumatoid arthritis
- chronic headache and facial pain—pain affecting the head and face
  eg. migraines, temporomandibular pain (TMJ)
- primary chronic pain—pain with no known physical origin
  eg. irritable bowel syndrome (IBS), fibromyalgia

Wise Words From a Client

"One step at a time. I will get there."

Doctors often use tests to eliminate possibilities as it relates to pain (Jacques, 2020). When all of the possible explanations have been exhausted, primary chronic pain is the diagnosis (Treede, R-D. et al 2015).

This diagnosis causes much distress for both patient and doctor. For the patient, they do not understand how their pain cannot be diagnosed. In the case of the doctor, the lack of diagnosis causes distress because they often wonder if something was missed.

Clients with primary chronic pain report feeling frustration with doctors and specialists and the healthcare system. As a result, they often utilize alternative therapies to find relief.

Finally, it is important to understand that pain can contain elements of multiple types of pain.

2.4 Be Clear About Your Goals

Consumers are looking to replace their medications with cannabis (Kvamme et al., 2021). Which types of medications can cannabis replace? Can it be done safely and effectively? We have witnessed many consumers successfully substitute their medications with cannabis.

Expert Tip

DO NOT alter any current treatment or therapies until you consult with your health-care provider.

It is important to develop a healthy and realistic understanding of cannabis use, while considering its effectiveness and safety.

Substituting Medications with Cannabis

First, let us consider the substitution of medications with cannabis.

A 2014 study compared states where medical cannabis was legal versus illegal. They found that deaths from opioid overdoses were substantially lower in states where medical cannabis was legal (Bachhuber, et al., 2014). A 2019 study by Shover et al. found that deaths from opioid overdoses had no discernible difference as described by Bachhuber (Shover et al., 2019). Researchers cannot validate whether cannabis has any effect on mortality rates due to opiate use.

A 2016 study looked at the prescribing habits of physicians where cannabis was legal for medical use. The findings saw the average doctor prescribing 1,800 fewer opioid doses per year to Medicare recipients. This study suggests that cannabis is contributing to a reduction in opioid prescriptions (Bradford, A.C., & Bradford, W.D., 2016).

Other studies suggest cannabis is replacing other types of medications. In addition to opioids, what types of prescriptions are people replacing with cannabis?

A 2017 study surveyed 2,774 people who reported having used cannabis in the previous three months. Almost half of those surveyed (46%) responded that they were using cannabis as a substitute for prescription drugs (Corroon Jr. et al., 2017). The most common substitutions were:

- opioids
- anxiety drugs
- antidepressants

The substitution of cannabis for pharmaceutical medications requires the consideration of many factors such as:

- You as an individual
- Your specific conditions
- Your experience with pharmaceuticals and their associated side effects
- Your experience with cannabis and its associated side effects
- The relief you experience from your chosen therapy
- Your overall treatment goals

Expert Tip

This is general information and not health advice about your specific medical condition. Discuss starting, stopping, or weaning off medications with your primary health-care provider. This is critical when deciding to substitute opioids for cannabis.

Understanding Symptom Management Versus Treating a Disease

Let us discuss the management of symptoms versus the treatment of disease. Symptoms are things you feel that relate to a condition, like "pain in my wrist." To manage symptoms means to reduce the effects of the underlying condition. In this example, managing the symptom would be relieving the pain in the wrist. Treating the disease involves halting, reversing, or slowing down the progression of an underlying condition. In this case, the therapy or treatment that actually reverses the condition would be what treats the disease.

Another example highlights these two concepts very well. In the treatment of rheumatoid arthritis, DMARDs (disease-modifying antirheumatic drugs) slow down the disease's process of tissue damage. In addition, opiates and anti-inflammatory medications can manage symptoms like pain and inflammation.

With all medications and treatments, it is always important to consider the risks of treatment versus the potential benefits. If a medication manages symptoms and treats disease, it is of maximum value. It will receive consideration as a therapy even if there are side effects. Again, it is a measure of risk versus benefit.

Cannabis has the potential to help manage symptoms of some conditions. A 2018 study found that cannabis can help manage depression symptoms, but does not improve the condition long term (Cuttler et al., 2018).

Chapter Summary

Chapter 2 provided the framework to gain clarity on your current state of health. This framework, gained through the Health Selfie, will serve as the foundation in developing your SMART health goal.

Be Clear Milestone

I am gaining clarity around my health by understanding where I am by completing my baseline assessments.

Chapter 3: Be Aware

Stage Characteristic

I am skeptical of the amount of information available online about medical cannabis and how it can relate to my needs.

3.1 Be Aware of Treatment Options with Cannabis

Cannabis is Not a One-Size-Fits-All Solution

Often, consumers share their successes with family and friends about how cannabis has helped their symptoms. However, what works for one may not work for another based on:

- genetics
- environment
- product variances
- method of consumption

There are many unfounded claims that suggest cannabis in general, and CBD specifically, can cure every problem that ails you. We want to make it clear that this is simply **NOT TRUE**. There are therapeutic qualities to both THC and CBD, but they do not help all conditions nor all people.

Limit Changes

When introducing cannabis, it is recommended to keep other therapies and medications as consistent as possible. The fewer things that change as you start your treatment, the easier it is to evaluate the response to your new therapy.

For example, if your doctor changed three medications at a recent visit, it would make no sense to start your cannabis treatment at the same time. It would be impossible to figure out what is responsible for the changes.

Keep things simple. Keep a journal detailing the way you feel. Self-awareness is a friend that you will develop as you progress on your path to wellness. The best results will come from your own cautious approach.

3.2 Cannabis and Mental Health

Anxiety and Anxiety Disorder

Anxiety is a normal part of life. Everyone experiences anxiety in certain situations. Think of your first day at a new school or job, or a time when you had to deliver a presentation. You would have experienced short-lived anxiety. Holland explains that anxiety disorders differ from anxiety in that they can be much more intense and/or frequent. They can cause severe levels of distress and fear, which interferes with one's ability to maintain their daily life. The anxiety connected with anxiety disorders lasts for at least six months (2020).

Some anxiety disorders include (National Institute of Mental Health, 2018):

- social anxiety disorder
- general anxiety disorder
- specific phobias

- panic attacks
- obsessive-compulsive disorder

There are many symptoms associated with anxiety. The Mental Health Commission of Canada describes some of the symptoms (2010):

- headaches
- tense, achy muscles
- restless legs
- upset stomach—nausea, vomiting, diarrhea
- sweats
- fatigue and exhaustion
- sensory overload
- shortness of breath, hyperventilation
- constant worry and stress
- difficulty concentrating
- trouble sleeping
- heart palpitations
- rapid heart rate

Although you may experience these symptoms at any time, it is important that you document these feelings and follow up with your primary care provider for a professional assessment.

Depression

The Centre for Addiction and Mental Health identifies depression as a mood disorder with symptoms described as:

- withdrawal from family and friends
- feeling worthless
- feeling hopeless
- feeling helpless
- guilt
- poor sleep
- mood swings

- suicidal thoughts
- changes in appetite or weight
- feeling tired all of the time
- loss of interest in activities that were once loved

Like anxiety, many people experience depression. Depression is a complex diagnosis that requires a professional assessment with your primary care provider. The presence of these symptoms does not mean you have depression. Your practitioner will likely rule out other causes or if any medications are responsible (Centre for Addiction and Mental Health, 2020).

Below are just a few conditions that may be mistaken for depression (Robinson, 2021):

- anemia
- chronic fatigue syndrome
- hypo/hyperthyroidism (low or excess thyroid function)
- anxiety disorders
- bipolar disorder
- substance abuse

Depression can be secondary to other conditions such as pain or sleep problems (Hall-Flavin, 2019). In some cases, treating the underlying cause of the pain or sleep issue actually resolves the depression without direct intervention. This is an example of why you should get a proper diagnosis from your provider before treating your depression.

Post-Traumatic Stress Disorder

The Centre for Addiction and Mental Health describes post-traumatic stress disorder (PTSD) as a disorder that occurs after the experience of a traumatic event. The traumatic event can cause actual or threatened harm (2020).

The National Institute of Mental Health describes some symptoms of PTSD (2020):

- re-experiencing the traumatic event
- dreams and flashbacks of the traumatic event
- difficulty sleeping
- withdrawal from things previously enjoyed
- feelings of blame, guilt or fear about the traumatic event
- avoidance of things related to the traumatic event
- angry outbursts
- feeling tense or on guard
- difficulty experiencing joy or happiness

Schizophrenia

The Centre for Addiction and Mental Health (CAMH) defines schizophrenia as a psychotic disorder that affects how a person thinks, feels, and experiences reality. Schizophrenia has what are called positive and negative symptoms. These do not mean good and bad. Positive means "in addition to" and negative means "absence or loss of" normal function (2020).

The American Psychiatric Association (APA) describes positive symptoms as hallucinations and delusions. Hallucinations are perceiving something that is not there. Delusions are false beliefs. Negative symptoms include loss of emotion, drive, or withdrawal (2020).

The Mayo Clinic, APA and CAMH describes other symptoms such as (2020):

- decreased concentration
- memory problems
- abnormal behaviour
- disorganized thinking and speech

Schizophrenia treatment includes medications and various therapies like cognitive-behavioral therapy. Treatment is lifelong, but early recognition and treatment can improve outcomes (CAMH, 2020).

Mental Health Conditions That Are Not Appropriate to Treat with THC

While anxiety, depression, and PTSD have studies showing some promise that cannabis may be helpful, this leads to an important discussion about mental health conditions that are not to be treated with THC based cannabis.

> ***Expert Tip***
>
> **Some mental health disorders should NEVER be treated with THC based cannabis.**

Some of these include personality disorders, bipolar disorder, and psychotic disorders like schizophrenia. If you recall a previous discussion on risk versus reward when giving medication, the same applies to cannabis. The risk versus reward for treating schizophrenia and these other disorders with THC is too stacked to the side of risk. We strongly advise against it. However, if you choose to pursue cannabis as a treatment, please do so under your psychiatrist's close supervision.

Does Cannabis Help Mental Health?

There are studies and research to support cannabis use for reduction of symptoms in anxiety, PTSD and depression.

The strongest support is in the treatment of anxiety disorders. CBD, THC, or a combination of both can reduce anxiety with the right treatment plan. Zuardi et al. found a "U" shaped dose response to CBD in anxiety for subjects who were public speaking. He and his colleagues found subjective measures of anxiety over public speaking were reduced in the group that received 300 mg, versus the other two groups that received 100 mg or 900 mg (2017).

From our experience, many consumers start with CBD, specifically for daytime symptoms. Some people do use THC, but the side effect of impairment limits its usefulness.

There is also evidence for the effectiveness of cannabis in the treatment of PTSD. The hypothesis in believing cannabis may be effective is that the areas of the brain affected in PTSD contain large amounts of cannabis receptors (Hill et al., 2018). In one study, cannabis reduced several symptoms of PTSD by more than half in the short-term, though there was no change in baseline symptoms over time (LaFrance et al., 2020).

There is evidence to support the idea that cannabis use reduces symptoms of depression in the short-term. However, it is unknown if cannabis is effective in the longer term (Li et al., 2020). Higher doses of THC should not be used in major depressive disorder (Sarris et al., 2020). It is important to work with your health-care providers to determine if this is the appropriate treatment or if there are effective alternatives.

It is our experience that people have successfully treated their stand alone depression symptoms. However, the greatest benefit to depression symptoms is when they occur concurrently with another condition. When that condition is treated, symptoms of depression ease.

Wise Words From a Client

"There will be brighter days ahead."

3.3 Cannabis and Sleep

Sleep Disorders

The National Institute of Health reports that 50–70 million Americans suffer from a sleep disorder (2006).

Pacheco (2020) describes sleep disorders as disruptions in normal sleeping patterns. The most common types of sleep disorders are:

- insomnia—difficulty in falling or staying asleep
- sleep apnea—characterized by periods of non-breathing while sleeping
- restless legs syndrome—a tingling or prickly sensation in the legs
- narcolepsy—the sudden and irresistible need to sleep during the day
- shift work disorder—disruption in the body's natural clock

Whatever the cause of the sleep disorder, lack of sleep can have a profound effect on you. Watson and Cherney (2020) include these effects:

- decreased physical performance
- impaired memory
- decreased alertness
- increased risk of accidents
- impaired attention
- moodiness
- increased tiredness
- impaired cognitive abilities

Often, consumers report side effects from sleep medications. As a result, many people substitute with cannabis to improve their sleep (Kvamme, 2021).

Gates discusses that heavy cannabis users have difficulty sleeping. There is no consensus on what type of cannabinoid to use for sleep: THC,

CBD, or both (2014). Consumers report successful treatment with various combinations of these.

Sleep Conditions Appropriate for Cannabis Treatment

Studies have shown that cannabis can improve the quality and duration of sleep. Cannabis may be be helpful when there is an underlying condition (Can You Use Cannabis for Sleeping?, n.d.).

From our experience, consumers report cannabis to be effective for insomnia. Insomnia can be acute or chronic, and treatment can vary based on several factors.

Santos-Longhurst describes acute and chronic insomnia. Acute insomnia is related to a specific short-term stressor. It could be related to a new job, the death of a loved one, illness, jet lag or short-term pain. Acute insomnia only lasts a few weeks. Difficulty sleeping at least three times per week and lasting more than three months is chronic insomnia (2018).

Difficulty falling asleep is described as onset insomnia while difficulty staying asleep is defined as maintenance insomnia (Pacheco, 2020). Both onset and maintenance insomnia can be chronic or acute.

Several studies have evaluated the effectiveness of cannabis and its effect on anxiety, PTSD, and insomnia with no conclusive results (Gates et al., 2014).

Sleep Disorders Inappropriate for Cannabis

Some sleep disorders should not be treated with cannabis. One example is sleep apnea. Sleep apnea can lead to heart attacks and strokes if left untreated (WebMD, 2021). This condition is characterized by periods of non-breathing, resulting in low oxygen levels while asleep. Often, sleep apnea is accompanied by snoring or waking up gasping for air (Suni, 2021).

Suni (2021) continues to describe other symptoms of sleep apnea as:

- getting up to urinate at night
- morning headache
- dry mouth

- irritability
- difficulty concentrating
- daytime sleepiness

There are two types of sleep apnea. Central sleep apnea occurs when your brain fails to tell your body to breathe, while obstructive sleep apnea results in your airway being blocked by soft tissue (Suni, 2021).

Obstructive sleep apnea is far more common and is often associated with snoring. With both types of apnea, people wake up feeling tired (Suni, 2021).

To diagnose sleep apnea, work with your primary care provider. Your provider may refer you to a sleep specialist to complete a sleep study. The sleep study takes place in a lab that monitors all facets of your sleep. A Continuous Positive Airway Pressure (CPAP) device may be prescribed by your provider. This medical device uses a mask to maintain pressure in your airway, keeping it open.

Expert Tip

Although cannabis and over-the-counter medications may help you sleep, it may not solve the underlying problem. Always consult with your primary care provider.

What is Sleep Hygiene?

Before introducing cannabis as a treatment option, there are some things you can do to improve your sleep.

The following tips are compiled from Suni and the Centers for Disease Control and Prevention:

- keep a sleep schedule
- create a bedtime ritual
- avoid naps in the afternoon
- exercise
- create a comfortable environment
- avoid caffeine
- light snack
- unplug electronics
- stop looking at the clock
- use a sleep diary

Incorporating regular sleep habits and good sleep hygiene can improve your sleep.

Helpful Resource

For more information on sleep hygiene, visit: mypathtobewell.com

3.4 Cannabis and Pain

Previously, we discussed pain and how it is classified.

- Chronic pain—present for six months or longer
- Acute pain—shorter in duration and often follows trauma

Chronic Pain and How it May Affect Other Parts of Your Life

Chronic pain is acute pain that has not gone away. Left unresolved, it can affect other parts of your life.

Ask yourself the following. Does pain:

- cause you to be irritable or depressed?
- affect your relationships with friends and family?
- affect your performance at work?
- affect your sleep?
- cause you to consistently wake up feeling tired?
- cause you to avoid activities that might make your pain worse?
- cause you to miss activities previously enjoyed?
- cause you anxiety?

As you answer yes to more questions, you may begin to see how pain is impacting your path to wellness. Follow up with your primary care provider for support.

How Cannabis Can Provide Relief

Chronic pain may be steady or it may come and go (Cirino, 2018). It could have elements of both. Examine your situation. Choose a pain control that matches the frequency and duration of your chronic pain.

Cannabis can be used to treat chronic pain. We typically recommend a method of consumption that provides long-lasting effects for pain that is there all the time. Some examples are capsules, edibles or oil administered under the tongue. Depending on what part of the body is involved, we sometimes recommend topical applications.

We urge you to take caution as it can be greater than thirty minutes to feel any effects. For pain that is intermittent and requires faster pain relief, inhalation may be a better option.

Clients relate to us that cannabis can be effective for breakthrough pain. Until further research is available, we may continue to see inconsistent results.

Chronic Pain Coexisting With Other Conditions

Chronic pain often exists alongside other conditions.

Dahan (2014) describes some of these as:

- depression
- anxiety
- sleep disorders
- fatigue

It is important to work with your health-care provider to ensure the proper assessment and management of all your conditions. We caution you to never stop or taper off any medication without the guidance of your primary care provider.

In summary, cannabis can help with many types of chronic pain. Consider long-acting cannabis when pain is present most or all of the time. Inhaled cannabis is fast-acting and can be useful in some circumstances. That said, there is not much research to support its effectiveness relative to alternatives for the treatment of breakthrough pain.

> ***Wise Words From a Client***
>
> **"After trying other treatments, I am eager to find the right solution for me."**

3.5 Cannabis and Autoimmune Conditions

Autoimmune Conditions

According to the National Institute of Environmental Health Sciences (NIEHS), there are at least eighty autoimmune diseases (2021). The

NIEHS' definition: "Autoimmune disease is where the body attacks its own tissues. In normal circumstances, the immune system is supposed to keep us healthy by attacking invaders like viruses and bacteria. In the case of autoimmune conditions, the body's immune system is overactive and mistakenly targets normal tissue and organs."

Here is a short list of the most common autoimmune conditions (Shomon, 2021):

- rheumatoid arthritis
- inflammatory bowel disease
- diabetes mellitus
- lupus
- multiple sclerosis
- psoriasis

Shomon continues, "Autoimmune attacks come and go. This means that there are periods of attack and remission. The immune system seems to retreat and rest for a while before attacking the body again. These intermittent attacks or flare-ups cause permanent damage." Limiting the frequency and severity of attacks can prevent permanent destruction of tissue.

Approximately 25% of people with one autoimmune condition develop a second autoimmune condition (Eustice, 2020). In cases like this, autoimmune conditions are capable of damaging tissue throughout the body.

Autoimmune Conditions and Stress

People with autoimmune conditions often fear the next attack. Attacks may be brought on by stress. The disease itself is quite capable of causing stress too. Attacks can be painful and disabling. Unfortunately, these attacks contribute to permanent damage and further disability.

Sharif et al. discusses the relationship between stress and autoimmune diseases. "Attacks may be brought on by stress. Studies have shown that stress can affect the onset or duration of autoimmune diseases. As you create a treatment plan, consider ways to reduce stress that may trigger the onset of another attack. There is evidence that stress reduction may reduce autoimmune disease activity" (2018).

How Cannabis Can Help With Autoimmune Conditions

Clinical evidence to support the role of cannabis in treating autoimmune diseases is slowly mounting. Many people with autoimmune disease use cannabis and feel that it helps. But, the best understanding of how cannabis helps comes from its effects on reducing inflammation.

There are a large number of cannabinoids present in the cannabis plant. Many cannabinoids are anti-inflammatory agents. Reduction of inflammation is an important goal in treating autoimmune conditions (Bandoim, 2021).

Turcotte (2016) found that cannabinoids reduce inflammation by:

- shortening the lifespan of attacking immune cells
- inhibiting the growth of new ones
- interfering with the production of inflammatory agents
- assisting the function of cells that regulate overactive immune responses

Cannabis may help people suffering from autoimmune disorders. Before attempting to treat autoimmune conditions with cannabis, consider your doctor's advice including the use of DMARDs. DMARDs (disease-modifying antirheumatic drugs) prevent the destruction of tissue. Cannabis, as an anti-inflammatory, may be an effective adjunct treatment.

It is important to work with your doctor and specialist, specifically when looking to incorporate cannabis into treating your autoimmune condition.

3.6 Cannabis and Alzheimer's, MS, and Parkinson's

Alzheimer's, Multiple Sclerosis and Parkinson's

Alzheimer's, multiple sclerosis and Parkinson's disease are all neurodegenerative diseases, meaning:

- neuro—having to do with the brain
- degenerative—having to do with degeneration or destruction.

These diseases cause brain tissues to deteriorate, resulting in a gradual decline in function.

The Alzheimer's Association describes Alzheimer's as a progressive disease. Scientists believe brain cells are starved, and over time this causes cells to die. When enough cells die, there are profound changes. Alzheimer's is the most common cause of dementia. A primary characteristic of dementia is memory loss (2021).

Multiple sclerosis (MS) is a progressive and disabling disease of the brain and spinal cord. Protective sheaths in nerve cells are damaged, causing dysfunction. Excessive fatigue is a symptom of nervous system damage, but is often viewed as laziness by others (Groetzinger, 2014). Individual symptoms may vary depending on the extent of nerve damage.

Pietrangelo (2020) and the MS Society of Canada (2020) discuss some other common symptoms of MS such as:

- difficulty walking
- numbness and tingling in the limbs
- pain
- spasticity
- bladder control issues
- weakness

Parkinson's is the second most common neurodegenerative condition following Alzheimer's (Erkkinen et al., 2018). Parkinson Canada describes Parkinson's as a progressive disease of the brain affecting movement (2021).

The article continues to describe some signs and symptoms of Parkinson's, including:

- tremors
- stiff limbs
- slow movements
- altered balance
- muscle rigidity

Alzheimer's, multiple sclerosis and Parkinson's have no known cures. It is important to work with your health-care provider to help slow disease progression as well as safely consider cannabis as an adjunct therapy. There is a growing body of evidence that cannabinoids may have neuroprotective properties (Maroon and Bost, 2018).

Cannabis and Alzheimer's Disease

Researchers and patients have begun to explore cannabis as a means to slow disease progression. Animal studies have shown preserved memory and reduced learning impairment (Aso et al., 2015).

A 2019 study looked at 178 patients across twelve different studies and found no relevant evidence-based use of cannabis in treating dementia. Further, the authors suggest that cannabis may be effective for treating associated symptoms but requires further study (Peprah et al., 2019).

Cannabis and Multiple Sclerosis

From our experience, many consumers affected by MS use cannabis to treat symptoms. There is evidence that cannabis can help with the spasticity associated with MS, although some patients also use it to treat pain, tremors, and bladder problems (Frontline Medical Communications Inc., 2013).

There are many medications that can reduce the number and severity of attacks and improve long-term outcomes for patients with multiple sclerosis (MS Society of Canada, 2021).

Cannabis and Parkinson's

From our experience, many consumers with Parkinson's disease use cannabis to treat symptoms. Clinical research on the use of cannabis for Parkinson's is limited. A survey of 339 people with Parkinson's using cannabis found that 46% indicated that cannabis produced some amount of lessening their symptoms (Venderová et al., 2004).

There is some evidence that CBD may alter the progression of some neurodegenerative conditions (Iuvone et al., 2009).

The limited research to validate the safe use of cannabis for Parkinson's is inconclusive. We urge you to work with your health-care provider and specialist to use proven therapies for your care.

> ***Wise Words From a Client***
>
> **"I have so much to gain."**

3.7 Cannabis and Seizures

What are Seizures?

Seizures can be characterized by involuntary movements. Alternatively, the seizure may result in limited awareness with abnormal behaviours. Whatever the type of seizure, the cause is abnormal nerve activity in the brain (Watson, 2019).

As stated by Zimlich (2021), seizures are caused by:

- fever
- low blood sugar
- a tumour
- stroke

- epilepsy
- trauma
- infection

How Can Cannabis Help With Seizures?

We strongly recommend extreme caution when considering any form of cannabis to treat seizures. From our experience, parents who have exhausted many treatment options find themselves seeking a solution. There is limited research available to support and validate cannabis use for the pediatric population. It is paramount that you work with your health-care team in deciding if cannabis is a safe treatment option. The safety of long-term cannabis use in children has not been established (Fasinu et al., 2016).

Interest in cannabis as a treatment for seizures has been growing. Devinsky et al. conducted a placebo-controlled trial of CBD in patients with severe forms of epilepsy. The study found the addition of CBD to regular anti-seizure medications resulted in decreased seizures (2018).

Although pharmaceutical medications can reduce the severity and frequency of seizures, many of these medications can produce undesirable side effects (Goldenberg, 2010).

In summary, seizures are caused by the uncontrolled firing of nerves in the brain. It is vitally important that a coordinated approach to care is done with your health-care team.

3.8 Cannabis and Autism

What is Autism?

There are links between epilepsy and autism (Wright, 2019). Healthline describes autism as a developmental disorder where social interaction is challenging. Behaviours may be abnormally repetitive. People with autism may have a restricted number of activities that interest them (2021). People with autism may have language delays and intellectual disabilities (Raising Children Network, 2020).

Preliminary research by Dr. Aran concluded that CBD can be a promising treatment option for autism (2018).

Much like seizure disorders, autism is thought to be the result of abnormal nerve connections and firing (Takarae & Sweeney, 2017).

3.9 Cannabis and Cancer

Can cannabis treat cancer? Can cannabis improve the outcome?

Before we address that, let us examine what we know about cannabis and cancer.

Chemotherapy-Induced Nausea

Cannabis can be an effective treatment for nausea and vomiting caused by chemotherapy. Traditional prescription anti-nausea drugs often cause negative side effects. There is research to support that cannabis can be effective at treating this form of nausea (Smith et al., 2015).

Types of Cancer Research

It is important to introduce the types of research as it relates to cannabis and cancer. Research runs through a progression of three types of studies:

1) in vitro—analysis of cells in test tubes
2) animal models—studies of animals and the way their systems work. Some animals have systems that function in a similar manner to humans.

One research example is that cannabinoids can inhibit the multiplication of cancer cells in animal models (Velasco et al., 2016).

Another study, which involved mice with pancreatic cancer, found those treated with an anti-cancer drug and CBD lived three times longer than those treated with an anti-cancer drug alone (Ferro et al., 2018).

These are preliminary studies only. Please remember these results do not automatically translate to humans. Use extreme caution and work with your health-care team if considering cannabis.

3) human studies—examination of effective treatment in an actual human.

There are large ethical considerations for this type of study. The human subject may receive something that could help them, do nothing, or even hurt them.

Research continues to find treatment alternatives for cancer-related symptoms. There are well-established cancer treatments that should not be dismissed in favour of cannabinoid therapy. Until research makes further breakthroughs in human trials, cannabis may be best as a treatment adjunct for symptoms related to cancer and its treatments, and not a cure.

3.10 SMART Goals

Every year, most of us go through a process of goal setting. Maybe it is to exercise more, cut back on sweets, or lose some weight. Many go through this ritual every January, but few succeed. Why is that?

Most often, we have ideas of what we want to achieve, but fall short. By breaking down a goal into smaller parts while being accountable, you can increase your chances at success.

This section is aimed at helping you set goals that are realistic and achievable. A common method is to establish a SMART goal.

What Is a SMART Goal?

According to MindTools (2021), a SMART goal is one that is:

- **S**pecific—It is exactly what you want to accomplish.
- **M**easurable—It allows you to monitor your progress.
- **A**ttainable—It is achievable.
- **R**ealistic—It is doable considering your current day-to-day life.
- **T**ime-Bound—Having an end in sight helps you to focus and push yourself.

Helpful Resource

To get a SMART goal worksheet, visit: mypathtobewell.com

Chapter Summary

Chapter 3 reviewed a range of medical conditions to help you gain clarity on your current state of health. People are often skeptical about the amount of information available and how cannabis may relate to their needs. Establishing a health goal that is focused on you is an important first step after you seek clarity with your health selfie. You will build upon this strong foundation as you move forward in creating a treatment plan.

Be Aware Milestone

I have set health goals that are important to me.

Chapter 4: Be Informed

Stage Characteristic

I do not want to get "high" and have many questions about methods of consumption with a health conscientious outlook. I am concerned with my doctor's response and reaction.

4.1 The Endocannabinoid System

The Endocannabinoid System and Its Receptors

There are many systems in the body. These systems oversee specific body functions. Some control hormones, some control blood vessels, and some control clotting. They all work without any conscious thought. In the 1990s, the Endocannabinoid System (ECS) was discovered (Pertwee, 2006).

Raypole (2019) outlines some of the functions of the ECS, including:

- sleep
- pain
- cognition (mood, memory, and learning)

- appetite
- movement and motor control
- inflammation
- cardiovascular system control

All systems strive for the same objective—balance. If something upsets that balance, there is a need to restore that balance. The ECS is responsible for restoring that balance.

Who Are the Players?

Every system in the body has receptors. They are like locks. When they open, things occur and action happens. This process is called stimulation.

In the ECS, the receptors are called Cannabinoid Receptors (CB1 and CB2). These receptors are present throughout the body. They can be found in the nervous system, spleen, immune system, digestive tract, liver, heart, and lungs (Kendall & Yudowski, 2017).

Every system in the body has something to stimulate its receptors. Often, they are referred to as keys. In the ECS, the keys are called cannabinoids. They stimulate cannabinoid receptors (CB1 and CB2). The body produces its own cannabinoids—called endocannabinoids. Alternatively, cannabis derivatives can provide the body with cannabinoids (Kendall & Yudowski, 2017).

Cannabinoids are actively regulating body functions. Restoring balance is the goal.

What Is This Balance?

Balance in biology is called homeostasis. Homeostasis is the ability to maintain stable internal conditions that are necessary for optimal health and well-being (Britannica, 2020). A significant function of the ECS is to maintain homeostasis (Raypole, 2019).

4.2 CBD

What Is CBD?

Cannabidiol (or CBD) comes from the cannabis plant. CBD does not produce the "high" and feelings of euphoria often associated with cannabis or marijuana. CBD does NOT bind to CB receptors.

How Does CBD Work in the Body?

Previously, we introduced receptors and how they operate like locks. When they open, action happens. We call the process of opening the locks *stimulation*. CBD does not open these locks, rather it interacts and causes a variety of responses.

An example of this CBD interaction can be found with the feel good neurotransmitter (anandamide—AEA). Known as the bliss molecule (Scherma et al., 2018), CBD prevents the elimination of it. By preventing elimination, CBD enables our bodies to use AEA more effectively (Leweke et al., 2012).

There are other CBD interactions. CBD can inhibit an overactive immune system. CBD can also reduce inflammation and pain (Nichols & Kaplan, 2020). Many clinical trials are currently underway to examine how CBD can help a variety of symptoms and conditions.

What Conditions Is CBD Appropriate For Treating?

The scope of this book is not to provide a list of conditions to treat with CBD. It is important to work with your health-care practitioner to establish a treatment plan with or without CBD.

From our experience, some reported therapeutic effects of CBD are:

- anti-inflammatory (analgesia)
- anti-seizure
- anti-anxiety
- antidepressant

- improved mood
- improved sleep

Side Effects of CBD

Many studies have shown that CBD has a good safety profile (Iffland and Grotenhermen, 2017). From our experience, there have been a small number of undesirable side effects reported while using CBD: dry mouth, diarrhea, and mild alertness or fatigue.

Expert Tip

Speak with your health-care practitioner before starting any CBD treatment. Both you and your clinician should understand the risk of taking CBD with your medicines.

CBD can present challenges if you are taking certain medications. CBD interactions can vary from benign to dangerous. This interaction often results in the other medication becoming more or less effective.

CBD blocks the breakdown of medications in the liver. In some cases, medications come to the liver to be broken down and eventually excreted. If CBD blocks this medication from being broken down, there will remain more medication in your body for a longer period of time (Harvard, 2021).

An example of a problematic interaction is with some blood thinners. CBD may increase levels of blood thinners, leading to an increase in the risk of serious bleeding (Devitt-Lee, 2015).

On the other hand, some medications start in the benign form and are broken down and activated in the liver. If CBD blocks activation of this type of medication, then the medication will not perform as intended.

An example of a dangerous interaction is the use of CBD with the cancer drug Tamoxifen. CBD reduces the effectiveness of Tamoxifen in the treatment of breast cancer (Parihar et al., 2020).

Helpful Resource

For more information on medication interactions, visit: mypathtobewell.com

4.3 THC

What Is THC?

Tetrahydrocannabinol (or THC) is generally the most abundant cannabinoid. It does produce the "high" and feelings of euphoria often associated with cannabis or marijuana. THC activates receptors of the endocannabinoid system, producing a variety of effects (Atakan, 2012).

Receptors located in the nervous system are responsible for the psychoactive effect of THC. Receptors located in the immune and gastrointestinal systems are responsible for the inflammatory response (Zou & Kumar, 2018).

Cells range between excited and restrained states. When in normal range, cells are in balance. Used at the right dose, THC can restore that balance. However, too much THC can cause an imbalance, leading to undesirable effects. THC as a treatment is all about restoring balance.

What Conditions Is THC Appropriate for Treating?

The scope of this book is not to provide a list of conditions to treat with THC. It is important to work with your health-care practitioner to establish a treatment plan with or without THC.

From our experience, some reported therapeutic effects of THC are:

- antidepressant
- anti-nausea
- anti-insomnia
- analgesic
- improve appetite

Side Effects and Complications with THC

THC can cause impairment and be addictive. Over time, high doses can decrease the user's motivation. THC can cause vomiting, low blood pressure, and increased heart rate (Canada, 2020). There are serious risks associated with THC use during pregnancy (Ryan, 2018). We always recommend speaking to your health-care practitioner before starting any THC treatment.

These complications may be dose-related, meaning higher doses pose more risks. However, it is important to be aware that these complications exist with any method of consumption (e.g., capsules, oil under the tongue, or smoked cannabis).

THC can interact with other medications, and it is important to work with your health-care provider in assessing any potential interactions (Antoniou, 2020).

Wise Words From a Client

"I know cannabis is my medicine, it helps me."

4.4 Minor Cannabinoids: CBN and CBG

The cannabis plant produces over a hundred different cannabinoids. Two of the better-known minor cannabinoids are cannabinol (CBN) and cannabigerol (CBG). Research continues to isolate and test many of these minor cannabinoids to identify therapeutic properties (Martinez, 2020).

Evidence does suggest that CBN is very sedating and can stimulate appetite. Preliminary research supports antibacterial, anti-inflammatory, and analgesic effects with less psychoactivity (Russo, 2011).

As of 2020, there are no studies that have tested the effects of CBG in humans. Animal studies suggest that CBG could play a role in treating inflammatory bowel disease, Huntington's disease, and produce antibacterial properties (VeryWell Mind, 2021). We caution our readers that these findings are lab studies only and not human trials.

4.5 Terpenes

What Are Terpenes?

Terpenes are compounds responsible for aromas found in most products. Terpenes are routinely added to household products such as soaps, shampoos, and deodorants. Products may contain terpenes to activate your senses and contribute to your experience. It has been suggested that cannabinoids may interact with terpenes to produce therapeutic effects (Russo, 2011).

What Are Some Therapeutic Effects of Terpenes?

Below is a list of common terpenes found in cannabis and their effects:

Terpene	**Where It's Found**	**Potential Effects**
limonene	lemons citrus peels	digestive aid anti-inflammatory antioxidant anti-stress (Sobel, 2019)
myrcene	hops lemongrass thyme mangoes	sedation muscle relaxation anti-inflammatory analgesia antioxidant (Russo, 2011)
pinene	pine trees rosemary	anti-inflammatory analgesia anti-anxiety antidepressant sedative protection against brain damage (Weston-Green et al., 2021)
linalool	lavender mint cinnamon rosewood basil citrus fruits	anesthetic analgesic relaxation calming (Białoń et al., 2019)

caryophyllene	black pepper rosemary oregano	anti-inflammatory immunomodulator cardioprotective neuroprotective gastroprotective (Hashiesh et al., 2021)
humulene	hops cloves ginger	anti-inflammatory (Rogerio, et al., 2009)
terpinolene	all spice essential oils citrus juniper	sedation anti-bacterial anti-fungal (Agus, 2021)
terpineol	lilac cajuput oil pine oil	antihypertensive antioxidant antiulcer (Khaleel, et al., 2018)

Helpful Resource

For more information on terpenes, visit:
mypathtobewell.com

The amount of terpenes varies from plant to plant. Studies continue to identify potential therapeutic effects of terpenes.

Linalool, often found in lavender, has been used for many years. In a controlled trial, linalool was shown to improve sleep in college students with insomnia (Lillehei et al., 2015). This suggests that cannabis strains high in linalool could have calming properties appropriate for sleep.

A review of more than a dozen studies suggested essential oils have a positive effect on sleep. Lavender was the most frequently studied. There were no adverse events reported (Lillehei and Halcon, 2014). Studies continue to explore the effects of terpenes, specifically in cannabis. Often consumers' response to their treatment can be related to terpenes.

What Is the Entourage Effect?

The Entourage Effect refers to the idea that whole-plant cannabis is more effective than isolated cannabinoids and terpenes. To date, there are no studies that support this effect.

4.6 Methods of Consumption: Edibles

Edibles are those food and drink products that contain cannabis or its extracts. Edibles can provide a discreet, convenient and pleasant taste experience. Food and drinks used to create edibles include chocolate, candies and soda beverages. Alternatively, edibles can be made at home.

Capsules are typically made by extracting cannabis oil through a manufacturing process. This results in a standardized dose.

How Do Edibles Work?

Edibles are consumed orally and processed in the stomach. Taking edibles with fatty foods may help with absorption (Zgair et al., 2016). Once processed, cannabinoids move through the bloodstream to target areas. The effects of edibles can vary. Noticeable effects may take as little as two hours and last up to twelve hours (Grotenhermen, 2003).

The twelve hour period of effects make edibles an ideal dosing method for people who need symptom relief for an extended period of time.

Edibles are a discreet alternative to smoking or vaping.

Disadvantages of Edibles

If you are considering edibles as a method of consumption, keep in mind there are a few problems associated with ingestion.

- bioavailability—refers to the amount of active ingredient available after absorption. For example, the bioavailability of CBD edibles is very low. Over 80% of CBD taken by mouth may not be available for your body to use (Roizman, 2020).
- psychoactive form—a unique problem related to THC edibles. From the stomach, THC is carried directly to the liver. The problem is that the liver converts THC into a more psychoactive form. This form of THC enters the brain much quicker and easier, leading to very strong psychoactive effects (Barrus et al., 2016). This does not make THC edibles a bad choice. However, it is a factor to keep in mind if you are considering this dosing method.
- homemade—batches of edibles can be inconsistent depending on the starting material, cooking time and temperature.

Cautionary Notes

It is important to start low and go slow with edibles. It is not uncommon for naive people who do not feel the effects of an edible to take a second dose. The first dose will typically start to produce significant psychoactive effects after three hours, and then the second dose will kick in. As a result, some wind up in the emergency department with extreme paranoia and even psychosis due to over consumption.

Edible products are responsible for the large number of emergency department visits related to cannabis over-consumption (Mammoser, 2020).

Expert Tip

Please, for your own safety, only use tested products that are legally sourced.

4.7 Method of Consumption: Topical Cannabis

Topical application involves the use of cannabinoids placed directly onto the skin.

Topical application of cannabis can be used to treat (Medical News, 2021):

- skin conditions like psoriasis, eczema, or acne
- muscle and joint pain

From our experience, clients have reported benefits of topical cannabinoids for neuropathic pain and general joint aches and pains.

Topical application effectiveness may be limited due to penetration. Arthritic joint pain in the hands may see greater benefit than hip joints which are deeper from the surface of the skin (Nitecka-Buchta et al., 2019).

Expert Tip

Use caution as THC can cause impairment when applied topically.

4.8 Method of Consumption: Sublingual Absorption

One way to take cannabis oil is through sublingual administration. This means putting cannabis oil under your tongue.

How to Calculate Your Sublingual Dose

Cannabis oil comes in a bottle, and you will need a measuring device to administer a dose. Common measuring devices used are eye droppers or a syringe. You will need to determine the volume (ml) to administer according to your prescribed dose (mg).

Your health-care provider will recommend a dose in milligrams (mg). Do not confuse the dose (mg) with the amount or volume (ml). Seek clarity in determining the appropriate dose and volume for your specific circumstance.

A calculator to help you determine the volume can be found at the helpful resource below. Dose supplied is found on the bottle.

Helpful Resource

For assistance in converting from mg (amount of medicine) to millilitres (volume of medicine), please visit: mypathtobewell.com

How Does Sublingual Dosing Work?

There is good blood supply to the mouth. Holding the cannabis oil under your tongue allows for absorption to occur.

According to MacCallum and Russo (2018), this is important because:

- access to the bloodstream is direct, bypassing the stomach and liver
- effects can happen quicker
- it increases the bioavailability
- it makes the dose more effective

Sublingual dosing takes effect in thirty to ninety minutes and lasts about six to eight hours (Canadian Pharmacist Association, 2021).

Expert Tip

Start low and go slow when starting or changing your dosing.

Benefits and Limitations of Sublingual Dosing

The following is a list of the benefits of sublingual dosing:

- precise dose
- repeatable dose
- long periods of relief
- low cost per dose
- discreet

The long onset of action does not help with conditions that need immediate symptom relief. Some examples are breakthrough pain, sudden onset of anxiety, or migraines.

4.9 Method of Consumption: Inhalation

Smoking Versus Vaping

The most common method associated with cannabis consumption is inhalation. One popular method of inhalation is smoking. Smoking cannabis involves combusting cannabis and inhaling it. When you burn cannabis, you get not only the medicine but some of the unwanted by-products of combustion.

Vaporizing involves heating cannabis, but not igniting it. This method releases cannabinoids in a vapourized form. Vaporizing reduces the risks that are produced by smoking. Both dry cannabis and oil-based formulations can be vaped (CAMH, 2019).

How Does Inhalation Work?

Cannabis smoke or vapor passes into the lungs when you inhale it. From there, it enters the bloodstream very quickly (Eadie et al., 2021).

Inhalation provides an effect within minutes and lasts about two to four hours. Very high blood levels of the medicine can be achieved this way, but with this comes the associated euphoria and impairment. In short, inhalation starts working much quicker than sublingual or edibles, and delivers a very high dose that lasts a relatively short time (MacCallum & Russo, 2018). The most prominent advantage to inhalation is breakthrough symptom relief.

Below is a list of disadvantages to inhalation as a consumption method (Huestis, 2007):

- difficult to measure
- repeatable dose is hard to obtain
- not discrete
- odour
- lung health

Wise Words From a Client

"I have confidence in my choice of treatment with cannabis."

4.10 Designing Your Treatment Plan

Your journey began by gaining clarity on your health selfie. This section will focus on designing a treatment plan that is aligned with your health goals.

Work with your health-care provider when developing your treatment plan, especially if you are attempting to reduce other medications.

Helpful Resource

To get a copy of the treatment plan template, visit: mypathtobewell.com

The following formula will assist you in developing a treatment plan. Fill in the blanks with a focus on your desired outcomes.

for my________________________________ (condition)
I want__________________________ (CBD, THC or a blend)
at____________________________ (time of day- e.g., bedtime)
consumed by_________ (ingestion, inhalation, sublingual, topical)

Chapter Summary

Chapter 4 reviewed cannabinoids and the methods of healthy consumption. Establishing a treatment plan focused on you is an important first step after you develop a SMART goal. You will build upon this strong foundation as you move forward in implementing your treatment plan.

Be Informed Milestone

I am now informed and have a clearer understanding of the types of cannabinoids and how I want to consume my cannabis. I now have a treatment plan that is focused on me.

Chapter 5: Be Progressing

Stage Characteristic

I have started my treatment with cannabis and begun to evaluate how it may help with my chronic condition. I hope I can find relief and have access to the right product when needed.

5.1 Talk To Your Doctor

Why Is It Important to Talk to Your Doctor about Cannabis?

Cannabis use has a stigma attached to it. Clients have reported that their doctor:

- "*doesn't believe in cannabis*"
- "*got upset*"
- "*was dismissive when asked about it*"

These reactions may cause people to self-medicate. From our experience, clients may be reluctant to disclose cannabis use to family, friends or their health-care provider. Despite the possibility of a negative reaction, your health-care provider should be aware.

CBD and THC have the potential to interact with many medications (Harvard, 2021). These include:

- antidepressants
- blood thinners
- cancer medicines
- heart medicines

Interactions between medications are very common. Doctors and pharmacists are trained to recognize interactions and adjust your treatment plan accordingly.

Expert Tip

For your safety, explore possible drug interactions with your health-care provider.

Why Your Doctor May Have Difficulty with Cannabis

There are a number of reasons why your doctor may have issues with cannabis as part of your treatment plan:

- knowledge—the cannabinoid system is a recent discovery
- research—gold standard research to support cannabis use is lacking
- stigma—cannabis is perceived as having a high potential for abuse with no acceptable medical use (Gabay, 2013)

A 2020 study of Canadian doctors identified cannabis related knowledge gaps. A knowledge gap is the difference between the doctor's current knowledge and what the doctor would like to know. Knowledge gaps indicate that doctors want to learn (St. Pierre et al., 2020).

Wise Words From a Client

"I am grateful for my doctor, who cares for me and helped me to decide on a responsible treatment plan that included cannabis."

5.2 How to Access Medical Cannabis

Advantages of Using a Government Regulated Provider

Cannabis is readily available from a multitude of sources. Access to medical cannabis varies by jurisdiction.

Pharmaceutical medications are produced to high safety standards. Although pharmaceuticals may have side effects, the medications themselves are pure and free of contaminants. They are produced to contain exactly what is displayed on the label. Legal cannabis producers aim for the same standard.

Regulated safety standards help ensure that cannabis is:

- of high quality
- free of impurities
- accurately labelled
- consistent between batches

Expert Tip

Purchase your cannabis from a regulated provider to ensure quality and safety standards are met.

Risks With Using an Unregulated Provider

Be aware of products that may seem legal but are not. They are found everywhere, especially on the internet, and they can be dangerous. Some black-market sellers have put lead powder in cannabis to increase the weight (and thus the price). The New England Journal of Medicine documented a series of lead-poisoning cases traced back to a source of contaminated cannabis (Busse et al., 2008).

Another issue with unregulated providers is labelling. A 2017 study found inaccurate labels in 70% of CBD products purchased online. These products contained significantly more or less CBD than was disclosed on the label, and 21% actually contained THC (Bonn-Miller et al., 2017).

How Quality Lab Testing Can Confirm Product Safety

Lab testing ensures cannabis is free from substances that can be harmful. Further, it validates that the product matches the label. Testing ensures that banned substances are not present.

To identify legal, medical-grade cannabis, you can look for the following (Canada, 2021):

- The product is third-party tested
- There is government oversight of the producer's operations
- The concentration of THC and CBD is clearly labelled on the container
- The producer provides you with a proper receipt

5.3 Calculating Cost

From our experience, many of our clients evaluate cost when considering a method of consumption. It can be difficult to figure out which method of consumption is going to give you the best value. Different units of measurement make this inherently difficult.

The following may help reduce the cost of your medicine:

- choosing a cheaper method of consumption
- considering dosing and titration
- comparing delivery devices
- comparative shopping
- private insurance
- group benefit plans
- government benefits
- tax exemptions on medical cannabis
- seniors discounts
- veterans discounts
- low-income discounts
- group or health coaching

Wise Words From a Client

"The cost of cannabis is an investment into my well-being."

To gain a better understanding of costs based on your method of consumption, see the chart below. Use the costs for your area as well as the amount you use if applicable.

Cost Analysis
Per Day and Per Month with Various Methods of Administration

Dry	*Cost*	*Grams*	*Cost per gram*	*Grams used per day*	*Cost per day*	*Cost per month*
Smoke	$70	10	$7	1	$7	$210
Vape	$70	10	$7	0.75	$5.25	$157.50

	Cost	*Mg*	*Cost per mg*	*Mg used per day*	*Cost per day*	*Cost per month*
Oil	$75	1,000	$0.08	20	$1.50	$45
THC Capsules	$34.95	300	$0.12	20	$2.33	$69.90
CBD Capsules	$64.95	450	$0.14	30	$4.33	$129.90
THC Spray	$40	312	$0.13	20.8	$2.67	$80
CBD Spray	$45	312	$0.14	20.8	$3	$90

Helpful Resource

To get a copy of the cost analysis worksheet, visit: mypathtobewell.com

5.4 How to Start Your Cannabis Dosing

Start Low, Go Slow and the Therapeutic Window

Cannabis dosing follows a *start low and go slow* mantra. This means starting a medication at a low or minimum dose and then slowly increasing as needed.

Starting medicines at a lower dose can:

- allow the body time to get used to the medication
- reduce side effects
- allow you to arrive at an optimal dose without taking too much medicine

The therapeutic window is the idea that a medication will produce therapeutic benefits in a dosing range. Too small a dose will produce no benefit. Too large a dose, the therapeutic benefit may decrease or undesired side effects may be present. The goal is to maximize therapeutic benefit while experiencing little or no side effects (McGraw-Hill, n.d.).

In a study of 263 opioid-treated cancer patients with poorly controlled pain, the group receiving 21 mg of combined THC and CBD each day experienced a significant reduction in pain levels. This reduction was greater than the group that received 52 mg daily. The group that received 83 mg daily reduced their pain no better than with a placebo, but experienced more adverse effects (Portenoy et al., 2012).

This study demonstrates an example of the therapeutic window for cannabis. Although cannabis is generally a safe medication, there appears to be optimal dosing. For example, using a small THC dose to treat anxiety can help a bit, but using too big a dose can make anxiety worse.

> ***Expert Tip***
>
> **Always start low and go slow when starting or altering your treatment plan.**

Safe Storage

There are some things to consider when storing your cannabis in a safe manner. Like other medications, it is imperative to store your cannabis in places that cannot be accessed by kids and pets. In the case of cannabis edibles, they should be labelled and stored to ensure that they cannot be mistaken for products that look similar.

Store cannabis in such a way to preserve the life of the cannabinoids. There are three things that can cause cannabis to break down quicker. These are light, oxygen, and heat.

For dry cannabis, store in a cool, dry and dark place. Be sure to keep it away from appliances that emit heat. The refrigerator can also speed up the breakdown process of dried cannabis (Ontario, 2021).

For cannabis extracts, store in a cool, dry, and dark place. The refrigerator is an ideal place to prevent cannabis extract breakdown.

5.5 Titration

What is Titration?

Previously, we discussed how to introduce a cannabis treatment. When introducing medications, there is an adjustment period. Often, clients tell us that the most undesired side effects they experience are related to THC and the associated feelings of impairment.

With the first administered dose of a medication, look for adverse reactions. Subsequently, watch for subtle side effects which may be uncomfortable.

Evaluate your cannabis treatment by asking:

- *Is it doing what I was hoping it would do?*
- *Am I where I want to be?*

Expert Tip

Starting and titrating your treatment plan should follow your health-care provider's recommendations.

Let us examine CBD as it is used to reduce pain.

1. "Is it doing what I was hoping it would do?"

Yes: There is some pain reduction, and you are moving in the right direction.

Go to question 2.

No: Consider taking more time or talking to your health-care provider regarding your options.

2. "Am I where I want to be?"

Yes: The correct dose is being taken. Congratulations, you have successfully titrated!

No: You may have to increase or decrease the dose.

These questions should be asked on a weekly basis to evaluate your current dose. A week allows your body time to become accustomed to that dose. It is important to keep a health journal to document your day-to-day response to treatment. This will assist in evaluating the dose. This slow, methodical process is important for your safety. However, safe titration does not mean that severe negative events cannot happen. It just means there is a reduction in the likelihood of these things occurring.

Helpful Resource

To get a copy of the Step by Step Guide to Titrating Your Cannabis Dosing, visit: mypathtobewell.com

5.6 Your Cannabis Journal

Health Recordkeeping

Have you ever gone to a doctor's office or the emergency room and been asked a series of questions and found that you were only able to answer a few? And for some of the other questions, you were struggling to come up with anything? This is where health recordkeeping comes in handy.

Your health record should include:

- medical diagnoses
- symptoms
- surgeries
- lab results
- medications
- allergies
- demographic information
- next of kin information

The health record should be updated as events happen. For example, if you went to the emergency room last week for an appendicitis, you would want to include that visit in your health record, plus any surgery (if performed) and the medications that you were prescribed.

Journaling

Journaling daily will help add clarity to your response to treatment. Using the previous example, let us say you had surgery and were sent home with antibiotics and painkillers. Your next few days of journaling might relate to the level of pain you feel and how the medications are helping you manage your symptoms.

This will allow you to become an informed patient. Your health-care provider will see you as a good historian. This means that when the health-care provider is trying to figure out what is going on, they can depend on the accuracy of your answers. This makes it much easier for the provider to detect issues, order tests and provide good care.

On the other hand, a poor historian is unable to answer basic questions. This results in a more difficult assessment.

Journaling enables you to keep track of events in chronological order. This will help you avoid recency bias, where all you can remember is a recent event. Your cannabis journey is no different.

Often in conditions like pain, you will be asked to scale it from 1 to 10 (quantitative) and describe how it feels (qualitative). Journaling allows you to keep track of the variations of your treatment plan. We recommend you update your journal daily, especially at the onset of your treatment.

While you are journaling, do not be over concerned with a bad day. Look at the whole picture. If you have a poor day while you are feeling better overall, you should probably dismiss it as a bad day. Focusing on these little negative details can derail all the improvements that you have made. It is only after several poor days that you should be re-thinking titration.

Helpful Resource

To get a copy of the Health Journal, visit:
mypathtobewell.com

5.7 Cannabis and Impairment

Jurisdictions have different laws, rules and policies regarding impairment due to illegal drugs, prescriptions, or alcohol. This book is not a substitute for the laws of your jurisdiction or the rules of your workplace.

CAMH's Lower Risk Cannabis Use Guidelines states, "Cannabis use impairs your ability to drive a car or operate other machinery. Don't engage in these activities after using cannabis, or while you still feel affected by cannabis in any way. These effects typically last at least six hours, but could be longer, depending on the person and the product used. Using cannabis and alcohol together further increases your impairment. Avoid this combination before driving or operating machinery." (2021)

MADD Canada states, "Many drugs impair one's ability to drive. Depending on the drug type, it can reduce alertness, alter depth perception, impair concentration and attention span, slow reaction time, and affect motor skills and visual function. Many people think driving under the influence of cannabis is risk-free, and that drivers on cannabis are more cautious and drive slower."

MADD continues, "But studies show that cannabis can have a negative impact on driving, including reduced concentration and attention span, slower reaction time, and an altered perception of time and distance. Driving studies (simulated and on-road) showed drivers had increased variability in lane position, following distance and speed after cannabis use. Cannabis also affected the drivers' ability to react to unexpected events, such as a pedestrian darting out onto the roadway." (2021)

Be Progressing Milestone

I am committed to my health goals and working on small wins that contribute to my treatment plan. Daily, I see progress by testing and refining while journaling my results.

Chapter Summary

Chapter 5 provided tools to implement your treatment plan aligned with your health goal. We discussed strategies to get the most out of your treatment while documenting your results. You will build upon this strong foundation as you move forward and compare and contrast your response to treatment.

Chapter 6: Be Well

Stage Characteristic

I welcome and accept where I am now. I have a vision of my future path to wellness. I now take an active role in managing my health care.

6.1 Be Healthy

Health

Health is often viewed as the presence or absence of a disease or disability. A widely accepted concept of health encompasses a more holistic approach of the individual when defining their health. The World Health Organization defines health as a "state of complete physical, mental and social well-being, and not merely the absence of disease or infirmity." (1948).

Wellness

The Global Wellness Institute defines wellness as "the active pursuit of activities, choices and lifestyles that lead to a state of holistic health." (2021)

Wellness is:

- spiritual
- emotional
- environmental
- financial
- intellectual
- occupational
- physical
- social

Wise Words From a Client

"I have a path to wellness that is centred around me."

The Wellness Wheel includes social determinants of health. These factors can influence your health outcomes (WHO, 2021). Let us look at determinants that can and cannot be modified.

Non-Modifiable (cannot be changed):

- biology
- genetics
- family

Modifiable (can be changed):

- income and social status
- employment
- education
- physical environment
- social supports and coping skills

- behaviour (healthy versus unhealthy)
- access to health services

Helpful Resource

For more information on the Wellness Wheel, visit: mypathtobewell.com

6.2 Medication Awareness

No Magic Pill

In Chapter 2, gaining clarity with your medications was part of your health selfie. Let us build on this clarity as part of your health and wellness.

Medication awareness helps us to understand that there is no magic pill or one-size-fits-all solution. This is true for all medications, including cannabis. Having a clear understanding of what you hope to achieve by taking a medication, while evaluating the side effects, is good medication awareness.

Medication Awareness

The first step in developing medication awareness is to understand why you are taking the medicine.

As stated by the Institute for Work and Health (2021), medications are prescribed for three reasons:

- **Primary**: to prevent a disease
- **Secondary**: to prevent complications of a disease from developing
- **Tertiary**: to treat a symptom of a disease and improve the patient's quality of life

Developing medication awareness while understanding which of the three reasons a medication was prescribed to you will allow you to better advocate for your health.

Helpful Resource

For more information on medication awareness, visit: mypathtobewell.com

Side Effects

In many cases, medications do cause side effects. These can range from uncomfortable to serious.

When discussing side effects with your doctor or pharmacist, you should be able to:

- describe the side effects clearly and concisely
- be clear about the time frame

Expert Tip

Abruptly stopping some medicines can be uncomfortable, extremely dangerous, or even life-threatening. Always consult your prescribing physician first.

6.3 Complementary and Alternative Medicine

What is Complementary and Alternative Medicine?

Conventional treatment refers to western medicine. Complementary medicine is when non-conventional therapy is used together with conventional treatments. When a non-conventional therapy is used in place of conventional medicine, we call it alternative. The defining characteristic is not the therapy itself, but how it is used (NCCIH, 2021).

As you gain confidence, it may be time to introduce complementary and alternative care. More than 30% of adults may consider non-conventional therapies (Barnes et al., 2004).

Some complementary and alternative therapies include, but are not limited to:

- chiropractic
- massage
- naturopath
- reiki
- physiotherapy
- essential oils
- teas

Some complementary and alternative practices have not been studied in well-designed trials. There may not be good evidence to prove their usefulness or benefit. In some ways, this mirrors cannabis. There are many reports by individuals of the benefits of cannabis for certain conditions, but there is a lack of official studies. This may be the same for some of these other therapies. But for both of these, further research is critical.

Wise Words From a Client

"I have health-care choices that enable me to achieve my health goals."

What Are the Risks?

If you are considering a new treatment, learn as much as you can about the safety of the therapy. We urge you to understand all facets of a treatment.

Some considerations and red flags when evaluating a therapy are:

- adequate oversight
- large up-front payments
- claims of miracle cures

Missing out on proven treatments for serious conditions may be the most significant risk of using complementary and alternative medicine.

What Are the Benefits?

Complementary and alternative medicine providers may have more time to spend with you than your medical doctor. This may allow for a more holistic approach to your treatment, taking into account your lifestyle, environment, and habits. Picturing these changes and how they may help as a whole may motivate you to make positive changes.

Complementary and alternative medicine providers often seek to uncover underlying issues. This approach lends itself to the relief of symptoms.

Expert Tip

Include your primary care practitioner in your complementary and alternative treatment plan. This supports a team-based approach to ensure your safe care.

6.4 Reflect On Your Health Journey

Wow! You are in the last section, and you have accomplished so much. You came in at your starting point, perhaps feeling overwhelmed, lacking knowledge, and not knowing exactly how to start, but you persevered, and here you are.

You have gained clarity about:

- your health selfie
- factors affecting your health
- medication records
- sleep
- mental health
- SMART health goals
- cannabinoids
- methods of consumption
- treatment plans
- working with your doctor
- cannabis cost analysis
- health journaling
- the Wellness Wheel
- complementary and alternative medicine

What Does This All Mean?

As you look back, we hope you have gained clarity on your chronic medical condition. Your journey does not end here—it's just beginning.

If there is a subject you wish to have more clarity on, go back to that section and read it again. Alternatively, you can further your journey by re-visiting chapters that were important or resonated with you.

Additionally, we have many free resources available to you because you purchased this book.

To make more progress with the support of a health coach, and to implement a customized health plan with tools, resources, a course and community, visit mypathtobewell.com

For the thousands who were suffering, frustrated and discouraged in finding a solution so that they can feel well, we want to thank YOU for trusting us to be your health-care partner. For those starting out on their health-care journey, we look forward to hearing your stories. We wish for you to have a life filled with better days ahead.

Be Well Milestone

Congratulations! You have made tremendous results with your goals. Now it is time to build on the progress you have achieved.

Glossary

AD	Alzheimer's disease
AEA	arachidonylethanolamide
2-AG	2-arachidonoylglycerol
APA	American Psychiatric Association
ASD	Autism Spectrum Disorder
CAM	complementary and alternative medicine
CAMH	Centre for Addiction and Mental Health
CB1	cannabinoid receptor type 1
CB2	cannabinoid receptor type 2
CBD	cannabidiol
CBG	cannabigerol
CBN	cannabinol
CNS	central nervous system
CPAP	continuous positive airway pressure
DMARDs	disease-modifying antirheumatic drugs
DSM-5	Diagnostic and Statistical Manual, 5th Edition
eCBs	endocannabinoids
ECS	endocannabinoid system
HD	Huntington's disease
IBS	irritable bowel syndrome

MADD	Mothers Against Drunk Driving
mg	milligrams
ml	milliliters
MS	multiple sclerosis
NIEHS	National Institute of Environmental Health Sciences
PHAC	Public Health Agency of Canada
PTSD	post-traumatic stress disorder
SMART	Specific, Measurable, Attainable. Realistic, Time Bound
TBI	traumatic brain injury
THC	tetrahydrocannabinol
TMJ	temporomandibular joint
WHO	World Health Organization

Citations and References

Autism

Aran, Adi, Hanoch Cassuto, Asael Lubotzky, Nadia Wattad, and Esther Hazan. 2018. "Brief Report: Cannabidiol-Rich Cannabis in Children with Autism Spectrum Disorder and Severe Behavioral Problems—a Retrospective Feasibility Study." *Journal of Autism and Developmental Disorders* 49 (3): 1284–88. https://doi.org/10.1007/s10803-018-3808-2.

Cherney, Kristeen. "What Is Autism? Symptoms, Causes, Tests, Treatment, and More." Healthline. October 10, 2021. https://www.healthline.com/health/autism.

"How Autism Spectrum Disorder Affects Learning and Development." Raising Children Network. July 5, 2020. https://raisingchildren.net.au/autism/learning-about-autism/about-autism/how-asd-affects-development.

Takarae, Yukari, and John Sweeney. 2017. "Neural Hyperexcitability in Autism Spectrum Disorders." *Brain Sciences* 7 (12): 129. https://doi.org/10.3390/brainsci7100129.

Wright, Jessica. "The Link Between Epilepsy and Autism, Explained." October 21, 2019. Spectrum | Autism Research News. https://www.spectrumnews.org/news/the-link-between-epilepsy-and-autism-explained/

Cancer and Chemotherapy

Ferro, R., A. Adamska, R. Lattanzio, I. Mavrommati, C. E. Edling, S. A. Arifin, C. A. Fyffe, et al. 2018. "GPR55 Signalling Promotes Proliferation of Pancreatic Cancer Cells and Tumour Growth in Mice, and Its Inhibition Increases Effects of Gemcitabine." *Oncogene* 37 (49): 6368–82. https://doi.org/10.1038/s41388-018-0390-1.

Smith, Lesley A, Fredric Azariah, Verna TC Lavender, Nicola S Stoner, and Silvana Bettiol. 2015. "Cannabinoids for Nausea and Vomiting in Adults with Cancer Receiving Chemotherapy." *Cochrane Database of Systematic Reviews*, November. https://doi.org/10.1002/14651858.cd009464.pub2.

Velasco, G., C. Sánchez, and M. Guzmán. 2016. "Anticancer Mechanisms of Cannabinoids." *Current Oncology* 23 (March): 23. https://doi.org/10.3747/co.23.3080.

Cannabis and Impairment

Centre for Addiction and Mental Health. "10 Ways to Reduce Risks to Your Health When Using Cannabis." *Canada's Lower-Risk Cannabis Use Guidelines.* September 10, 2021. https://www.camh.ca/-/media/files/pdfs---reports-and-books---research/canadas-lower-risk-guidelines-cannabis-pdf.pdf

MADD. Mothers Against Drunk Driving. "Cannabis and Driving." September 10, 2021. https://madd.ca/pages/impaired-driving/overview/cannabis-and-driving/#3

Complementary and Alternative Medicine

National Center for Complementary and Integrative Health. 2021. "Complementary, Alternative, or Integrative Health: What's in a Name?" NCCIH. April 2021. https://www.nccih.nih.gov/health/complementary-alternative-or-integrative-health-whats-in-a-name.

Barnes, Patricia M, Barbara Bloom, Richard L Nahin, and National Center. *Complementary and Alternative Medicine Use among Adults and Children: United States, 2002*. Hyattsville, Md: Dept. Of Health and Human Services, Centers for Disease Control and Prevention, National Center for Health Statistics. 1-19. PMID: 15188733.

Depression

"Depression." CAMH. July 13, 2020. https://www.camh.ca/en/health-info/mental-illness-and-addiction-index/depression.

Flavin. "Depression Can Cause Pain—and Pain Can Cause Depression." Mayo Clinic. 2019. https://www.mayoclinic.org/diseases-conditions/depression/expert-answers/pain-and-depression/faq-20057823.

Robinson, K.M. "Things That May Look Like Depression But Aren't." WebMD. September 10, 2021. https://www.webmd.com/depression/looks-like-depression-but-not

Edibles

Barrus, Daniel, Kristen Capogrossi, Sheryl Cates, Camille Gourdet, Nicholas Peiper, Scott Novak, Timothy Lefever, and Jenny Wiley. 2016. "Tasty THC: Promises and Challenges of Cannabis Edibles." 2016. https://doi.org/10.3768/rtipress.2016.op.0035.1611.

Grotenhermen, Franjo. "Pharmacokinetics and Pharmacodynamics of Cannabinoids." *Clinical Pharmacokinetics* 42 (4): 327–60. 2003. https://doi.org/10.2165/00003088-200342040-00003.

Mammoser, G. (2020, January 13). "Cannabis Edibles Aren't as Safe as People Think." January 5, 2021. https://www.healthline.com/health-news/cannabis-edibles-health-risks

Roizman, T. "CBD Bioavailability: What Does It Mean Why is it so Important?" Daily CBD. November 19, 2020. https://dailycbd.com/en/cbd-bioavailability/

Zgair, A., et al. "Dietary fats and pharmaceutical lipid excipients increase systemic exposure to orally administered cannabis and cannabis-based medicines." *American Journal of Translational Research.* 2016. 8(8), 3448–3459.

Endocannabinoid

Britannica. "Homeostasis | Definition, Examples, & Facts." *Encyclopedia Britannica.* December 1, 2021. https://www.britannica.com/science/homeostasis.

Kendall, Debra A., and Guillermo A. Yudowski. "Cannabinoid Receptors in the Central Nervous System: Their Signaling and Roles in Disease." *Frontiers in Cellular Neuroscience.* 2017. https://doi.org/10.3389/fncel.2016.00294.

Pertwee, R.G. "Cannabinoid Pharmacology: The First 66 Years." *British Journal of Pharmacology.* 147: S163-S171. 2006. https://doi.org/10.1038/sj.bjp.0706406

Raypole, C. "A Simple Guide to the Endocannabinoid System." August 12, 2020. https://www.healthline.com/health/endocannabinoid-system

How to Access Medical Cannabis

Bonn-Miller, Marcel O, Mallory Loflin, Brian Thomas, Jahan Marcu, Travis Hyke, and Ryan Vandrey. "Labeling Accuracy of Cannabidiol Extracts Sold Online." *JAMA* 318 (17): 1708–9. 2017. https://doi.org/10.1001/jama.2017.11909

Busse, Franziska P., Georg Martin Fiedler, Alexander Leichtle, Helmut Hentschel, and Michael Stumvoll. "Lead Poisoning due to Adulterated Marijuana in Leipzig." *Deutsches Aerzteblatt Online.* 2008. https://doi.org/10.3238/arztebl.2008.0757

Public Safety Canada. "Buying Cannabis Online—What You Need to Know." January 18, 2021. https://www.publicsafety.gc.ca/cnt/cntrng-crm/llct-drgs/llgl-nln-sls-cnnbs-en.aspx

How to Start Your Cannabis Dosing

Portenoy, Russell K., Elena Doina Ganae-Motan, Silvia Allende, Ronald Yanagihara, Lauren Shaiova, Sharon Weinstein, Robert McQuade, Stephen Wright, and Marie T. Fallon. "Nabiximols for Opioid-Treated Cancer Patients with Poorly-Controlled Chronic Pain: A Randomized, Placebo-Controlled, Graded-Dose Trial." *The Journal of Pain: Official Journal of the American Pain Society* 13 (5): 438–49. May 2012. https://doi.org/10.1016/j.jpain.2012.01.003.

"Therapeutic Window." n.d. TheFreeDictionary.com. September 7, 2021. https://medical-dictionary.thefreedictionary.com/therapeutic+window.

How to Talk to Your Doctor

Gabay, Michael. "The Federal Controlled Substances Act: Schedules and Pharmacy Registration." *Hospital Pharmacy* 48 (6): 473–74. 2013. https://doi.org/10.1310/hpj4806-473

ScD, Katsiaryna Bykov, PharmD. "CBD and Other Medications: Proceed with Caution." *Harvard Health Blog.* December 3, 2021. https://www.health.harvard.edu/blog/cbd-and-other-medications-proceed-with-caution-2021011121743.

St Pierre, Michelle, Liam Matthews, and Zach Walsh. "Cannabis Education Needs Assessment among Canadian Physicians-In-Training."

Complementary Therapies in Medicine 49 (March): 102328. 2020. https://doi.org/10.1016/j.ctim.2020.102328

Medicinal Cannabis

Ryz, Natasha R., David J. Remillard, and Ethan B. Russo. "Cannabis Roots: A Traditional Therapy with Future Potential for Treating Inflammation and Pain." *Cannabis and Cannabinoid Research* 2 (1): 210–16. 2017. https://doi.org/10.1089/can.2017.0028

Pain

Bachhuber, Marcus A, Brendan Saloner, Chinazo O Cunningham, and Colleen L Barry. "Medical Cannabis Laws and Opioid Analgesic Overdose Mortality in the United States, 1999-2010." *JAMA Internal Medicine* 174 (10): 1668–73. 2014. https://doi.org/10.1001/jamainternmed.2014.4005.

Bradford, Ashley C., and W. David Bradford. "Medical Marijuana Laws Reduce Prescription Medication Use in Medicare Part D." *Health Affairs* 35 (7): 1230–36. 2016. https://doi.org/10.1377/hlthaff.2015.1661

Corroon, Jamie, Laurie Mischley, and Michelle Sexton. "Cannabis as a Substitute for Prescription Drugs – a Cross-Sectional Study." *Journal of Pain Research* Volume 10 (May): 989–98. 2017. https://doi.org/10.2147/jpr.s134330

Cuttler, Carrie, Alexander Spradlin, and Ryan J. McLaughlin. "A Naturalistic Examination of the Perceived Effects of Cannabis on Negative Affect." *Journal of Affective Disorders* 235 (August): 198–205. 2018. https://doi.org/10.1016/j.jad.2018.04.054

Jacques, Erica. "How Your Doctor Makes a Chronic Pain Diagnosis." Very Well Health. December 10, 2021. https://www.verywellhealth.com/how-your-doctor-makes-a-chronic-pain-diagnosis-2564452

Kvamme, S.L., Pedersen, M.M., Rømer Thomsen, K. *et al.* "Exploring the Use of Cannabis as a Substitute for Prescription Drugs in a Convenience Sample." *Harm Reduct J* 18, 72. 2021. https://doi.org/10.1186/s12954-021-00520-5

Mastroianni, Brian. "Why Do Most Patients Use Medical Marijuana? Chronic Pain." Healthline. February 21, 2019. https://www.healthline.com/health-news/what-drives-patients-to-us e-medical-marijuana-chronic-pain

Rath, Linda. "The Connection Between Pain and Your Brain." Arthritis Foundation. December 3, 2021. https://www.arthritis.org/health-wellness/healthy-living/managing-pain/understanding-pain/pain-brain-connection

Santos-Longhurst, Adrienne. "Types of Pain: Classifications and Examples to Help Describe Your Pain." Healthline. November 20, 2021. https://www.healthline.com/health/types-of-pain

Shover, Chelsea L., Corey S. Davis, Sanford C. Gordon, and Keith Humphreys. "Association between Medical Cannabis Laws and Opioid Overdose Mortality Has Reversed over Time." *Proceedings of the National Academy of Sciences* 116 (26): 12624–26. June, 2019. https://doi.org/10.1073/pnas.1903434116

Treede, Rolf-Detlef, Winfried Rief, Antonia Barke, Qasim Aziz, Michael I. Bennett, Rafael Benoliel, Milton Cohen, et al. "A Classification of Chronic Pain for ICD-11." *PAIN* 156 (6): 1003–7. 2015. https://doi.org/10.1097/j.pain.0000000000000160

Anxiety

Holland, Kimberly. "Everything You Need to Know About Anxiety." Healthline. June 28, 2021. https://www.healthline.com/health/anxiety

Mental Health Commission of Canada. *Mental Health First Aid: Canada*. Sec 4: p.2. 2010.

The National Institute of Mental Health. "Anxiety Disorders." December 14, 2021. https://www.nimh.nih.gov/health/topics/anxiety-disorders#part_2235

Mental Health

Mental Health Commission of Canada. *Mental Health First Aid: Canada*. Ottawa: Mental Health Commission of Canada. Sec 1: p.1. 2011.

Public Health Agency of Canada. "Mental Health Promotion: Promoting Mental Health Means Promoting the Best of Ourselves." December 14, 2021. https://www.canada.ca/en/public-health/services/health-promotion/mental-health/mental-health-promotion.html

Truschel, Jessica. "Depression Definition and DSM-5 Diagnostic Criteria." December 9, 2021. https://www.psycom.net/depression-definition-dsm-5-diagnostic-criteria/

Method of Consumption—Inhalation

CAMH. Centre for Addiction and Mental Health. "Canada's Lower-Risk Cannabis Use Guidelines." November 5, 2021. https://www.canada.ca/content/dam/themes/health/carousel/LRCUG%20Evidence%20Brief%20Final%20English%20v2.pdf

Eadie, Lauren, Lindsay A. Lo, April Christiansen, Jeffrey R. Brubacher, Alasdair M. Barr, William J. Panenka, and Caroline A. MacCallum. 2021. "Duration of Neurocognitive Impairment with Medical Cannabis Use: A Scoping Review." *Frontiers in Psychiatry* 12 (March). March 12, 2021. https://doi.org/10.3389/fpsyt.2021.638962

Huestis M. A. "Human Cannabinoid Pharmacokinetics." *Chemistry & Biodiversity*. 4(8), 1770–1804. 2007. https://doi.org/10.1002/cbdv.200790152

MacCallum, Caroline A., and Ethan B. Russo. 2018. "Practical Considerations in Medical Cannabis Administration and Dosing." *European Journal of Internal Medicine* 49 (March): 12–19. 2018. https://doi.org/10.1016/j.ejim.2018.01.004

Method of Consumption—Sublingual

"How to Help Patients Find a Safe and Effective Dose." n.d. Canadian Pharmacist Assocation. November 18, 2021. https://www.pharmacists.ca/cpha-ca/assets/File/education-practice-resources/Cannabis%20Dosing%20and%20Titrating%20Final_web.pdf.

MacCallum, Caroline A., and Ethan B. Russo. "Practical Considerations in Medical Cannabis Administration and Dosing." *European Journal of Internal Medicine* 49 (March): 12–19. 2018. https://doi.org/10.1016/j.ejim.2018.01.004

Method of Consumption—Topical

Medical News Today. "CBD skin cream: How to use and best options." Medical News Today. December 10, 2021. https://www.medicalnewstoday.com/articles/cbd-skin-cream

Nitecka-Buchta, Aleksandra, Anna Nowak-Wachol, Kacper Wachol, Karolina Walczyńska-Dragon, Paweł Olczyk, Olgierd Batoryna, Wojciech Kempa, and Stefan Baron. "Myorelaxant Effect of Transdermal Cannabidiol Application in Patients with TMD: A Randomized, Double-Blind Trial." *Journal of Clinical Medicine* 8 (11): 1886. 2019. https://doi.org/10.3390/jcm8111886.

Minor Cannabinoids: CBN & CBG

Martínez, V., Iriondo De-Hond, A., Borrelli, F., Capasso, R., Del Castillo, M. D., & Abalo, R. "Cannabidiol and Other Non-Psychoactive Cannabinoids for Prevention and Treatment of Gastrointestinal Disorders: Useful Nutraceuticals?" *International Journal of Molecular Sciences.* 21(9), 3067. 2020. https://doi.org/10.3390/ijms21093067

Russo E. B. "Taming THC: Potential Cannabis Synergy and Phytocannabinoid-terpenoid Entourage Effects." *British Journal of Pharmacology.* 163(7), 1344–1364. 2011. https://doi.org/10.1111/j.1476-5381.2011.01238.x

"What is Cannabigerol (CBG)?" Very Well Mind. December 17, 2021. https://www.verywellmind.com/cannabigerol-cbg-uses-and-benefits-5085266

PTSD

"Post-Traumatic Stress Disorder." NIH Publication No. 20-MH-8124. August 10, 2021. https://www.nimh.nih.gov/health/publications/post-traumatic-stress-disorder-ptsd

"Post-traumatic Stress Disorder." The Centre for Addiction and Mental Health. July 16, 2020. https://www.camh.ca/en/health-info/mental-illness-and-addiction-index/posttraumatic-stress-disorder

Safe Storage

"How to Properly Store Cannabis." Ontario Cannabis Store. November 14, 2021. https://ocs.ca/blogs/cannabis-how-tos/how-to-properly-store-cannabis

Schizophrenia

"Schizophrenia—Symptoms and Causes." Mayo Clinic. July 17, 2020. https://www.mayoclinic.org/diseases-conditions/schizophrenia/symptoms-causes/syc-20354443

"Schizophrenia." The Centre for Addiction and Mental Health. July 17, 2020. https://www.camh.ca/en/health-info/mental-illness-and-addiction-index/schizophrenia

"What is Schizophrenia?" American Psychiatric Association. July 19, 2020. https://www.psychiatry.org/patients-families/schizophrenia/what-is-schizophrenia

Mental Health Studies

Hill, Matthew N, Patrizia Campolongo, Rachel Yehuda, and Sachin Patel. 2017. "Integrating Endocannabinoid Signaling and Cannabinoids into the Biology and Treatment of Posttraumatic Stress Disorder." *Neuropsychopharmacology* 43 (1): 80–102. https://doi.org/10.1038/npp.2017.162.

Li, X., Diviant, J. P., Stith, S. S., Brockelman, F., Keeling, K., Hall, B., & Vigil, J. M. "The Effectiveness of Cannabis Flower for Immediate Relief from Symptoms of Depression." *The Yale Journal of Biology and Medicine* 93(2), 251–264. 2020.

Sarris, Jerome, Justin Sinclair, Diana Karamacoska, Maggie Davidson, and Joseph Firth. 2020. "Medicinal Cannabis for Psychiatric Disorders: A Clinically-Focused Systematic Review." *BMC Psychiatry* 20 (1). January 16, 2020. https://doi.org/10.1186/s12888-019-2409-8.

"Short and Long-Term Effects of Cannabis on Symptoms of Post-Traumatic Stress Disorder." 2020. *Journal of Affective Disorders* 274 (September): 298–304. https://doi.org/10.1016/j.jad.2020.05.132.

Zuardi, Antonio W., Natália P. Rodrigues, Angélica L. Silva, Sandra A. Bernardo, Jaime E. C. Hallak, Francisco S. Guimarães, and José A. S. Crippa. 2017. "Inverted U-Shaped Dose-Response Curve of the Anxiolytic Effect of Cannabidiol during Public Speaking in Real Life." *Frontiers in Pharmacology* 8 (May). https://doi.org/10.3389/fphar.2017.00259.

Seizures

Devinsky, Orrin, Anup D. Patel, J. Helen Cross, Vicente Villanueva, Elaine C. Wirrell, Michael Privitera, Sam M. Greenwood, et al. "Effect of Cannabidiol on Drop Seizures in the Lennox–Gastaut Syndrome." *New England Journal of Medicine* 378 (20): 1888–97. 2018. https://doi.org/10.1056/nejmoa1714631

"Epilepsy vs. Seizures: Understanding the Difference." 2021. Healthline. February 25, 2021. https://www.healthline.com/health/epilepsy/epilepsy-vs-seizure

Fasinu, Pius S., Sarah Phillips, Mahmoud A. ElSohly, and Larry A. Walker. "Current Status and Prospects for Cannabidiol Preparations as New Therapeutic Agents." *Pharmacotherapy* 36 (7): 781–96. 2016. https://doi.org/10.1002/phar.1780.

Goldenberg, Marvin M. 2010. "Overview of Drugs Used for Epilepsy and Seizures: Etiology, Diagnosis, and Treatment." *P & T: A Peer-Reviewed Journal for Formulary Management* 35 (7): 392–415. September 5, 2021. https://www.ncbi.nlm.nih.gov/pmc/articles/PMC2912003/.

Watson, Stephanie. 2014. "The Effects of Epilepsy on the Body." Healthline. 2014. https://www.healthline.com/health/epilepsy/effects-on-body.

Sleep Disorders

"7 Ways Sleep Apnea Can Hurt Your Health." WebMD. January 12, 2011. Retrieved December 1, 2021. https://www.webmd.com/sleep-disorders/sleep-apnea/sleep-apnea-conditions

"Can You Use Cannabis for Sleeping?" Www.medicalnewstoday.com. August 31, 2018. Retrieved December 9, 2021. https://www.medicalnewstoday.com/articles/322945#does-cannabis-help-with-sleep

Gates, Peter J., Lucy Albertella, and Jan Copeland. "The Effects of Cannabinoid Administration on Sleep: A Systematic Review of Human Studies." *Sleep Medicine Reviews* 18 (6): 477–87. 2014. https://doi.org/10.1016/j.smrv.2014.02.005

Healthline. "11 Effects of Sleep Deprivation on Your Body." Healthline. May 15, 2020. https://www.healthline.com/health/sleep-deprivation/effects-on-body.

Institute of Medicine (US) Committee on Sleep Medicine and Research. *Sleep Disorders and Sleep Deprivation: An Unmet Public Health Problem.* Edited by Harvey R. Colten and Bruce M. Altevogt. *PubMed.* Washington (DC): National Academies Press (US). 2006. https://www.ncbi.nlm.nih.gov/books/NBK19960/

Kvamme, Sinikka L., Michael M. Pedersen, Kristine Rømer Thomsen, and Birgitte Thylstrup. "Exploring the Use of Cannabis as a Substitute for Prescription Drugs in a Convenience Sample." *Harm Reduction Journal* 18 (1). 2021. https://doi.org/10.1186/s12954-021-00520-5.

Santos-Longhurst, A. "What Is Chronic Insomnia and How Is It Treated?" Healthline. 2018. https://www.healthline.com/health/chronic-insomnia

Sleep Foundation. "Sleep Disorders | National Sleep Foundation." Sleepfoundation.org. 2019. https://www.sleepfoundation.org/sleep-disorders.

Suni, E. "Healthy Sleep Tips." Sleep Foundation. November 18, 2021. https://www.sleepfoundation.org/sleep-hygiene

Suni, E. "Sleep Apnea: What Is It, Its Risk Factors, Its Health Impacts, and How It Can Be Treated." Sleep Foundation. Retrieved July 9, 2021. https://www.sleepfoundation.org/sleep-apnea

"Tips for Better Sleep." Centers for Disease Control and Prevention. Retrieved July 15, 2020. https://www.cdc.gov/sleep/about_sleep/sleep_hygiene.html

Pain

Cirino, E. "What Causes Chronic Pain?" Healthline. Retrieved December 16, 2021. https://www.healthline.com/health/chronic-pain

Dahan, A., van Velzen, M. & Niesters, M. "Comorbidities and the Complexities of Chronic Pain." *Anesthesiology* 2014; 121:675–677. https://doi.org/10.1097/ALN.0000000000000402

Auto-Immune

Bandoim, L. "How Autoimmune Diseases Are Treated." Very Well Health. Retrieved October 4, 2021. https://www.verywellhealth.com/how-autoimmune-diseases-are-treated-5093794

Eustice, C. "What is Multiple Autoimmune Syndrome? Co-Occurrence of Autoimmune Diseases." Very Well Health. Retrieved December 16, 2021. https://www.verywellhealth.com/what-is-multiple-autoimmune-syndrome-4138360

National Institute of Environmental Health Sciences. "Autoimmune Diseases." Retrieved December 16, 2021. https://www.niehs.nih.gov/health/topics/conditions/autoimmune/index.cfm

Sharif, Kassem, Abdulla Watad, Louis Coplan, Benjamin Lichtbroun, Alec Krosser, Michael Lichtbroun, Nicola Luigi Bragazzi, Howard Amital, Arnon Afek, and Yehuda Shoenfeld. 2018. "The Role of Stress in the Mosaic of Autoimmunity: An Overlooked Association." *Autoimmunity Reviews* 17 (10): 967–83. 2018. https://doi.org/10.1016/j.autrev.2018.04.005

Shomon, M. "What Are Autoimmune Diseases?" Very Well Health. Retrieved December 16, 2021. https://www.verywellhealth.com/autoimmune-diseases-overview-3232654

Turcotte, Caroline, Marie-Renée Blanchet, Michel Laviolette, and Nicolas Flamand. "The CB2 Receptor and Its Role as a Regulator of Inflammation." *Cellular and Molecular Life Sciences* 73 (23): 4449–70. 2016. https://doi.org/10.1007/s00018-016-2300-4

Alzheimer's, Multiple Sclerosis and Parkinson's

Alzheimer's Association. "What Is Alzheimer's Disease?" July 10, 2020. https://www.alz.org/alzheimers-dementia/what-is-alzheimers

Aso E, Sánchez-Pla A, Vegas-Lozano E, Maldonado R, Ferrer I. "Cannabis-based Medicine Reduces Multiple Pathological Processes in AβPP/PS1 Mice." J Alzheimers Dis. 2015;43(3):977-91. doi: 10.3233/JAD-141014. PMID: 25125475.

"Disease-modifying Therapies." MS Society. July 11, 2020. https://mssociety.ca/managing-ms/treatments/medications/disease-modifying-therapies-dmts

Erkkinen, M. G., Kim, M. O., & Geschwind, M. D. "Clinical Neurology and Epidemiology of the Major Neurodegenerative Diseases."

Cold Spring Harbor Perspectives in Biology 10(4), a033118. 2018. https://doi.org/10.1101/cshperspect.a033118

Frontline Medical Communications Inc. "How Effective Is Marijuana for MS?" *Neurology Reviews.* 21(10):1, 25. MDedge Multiple Sclerosis Hub. October 2013. https://www.mdedge.com/multiplesclerosishub/article/77919/multiple-sclerosis/how-effective-marijuana-ms

Groetzinger, D. "Multiple Sclerosis: Its Effects on You and Those You Love." Multiple Sclerosis Society of Canada. July 12, 2020. https://mssociety.ca/uploads/files/2014-ms-effects.pdf

Iuvone, T., Esposito, G., De Filippis, D., Scuderi, C., & Steardo, L. "Cannabidiol: a Promising Drug for Neurodegenerative Disorders?" *CNS Neuroscience & Therapeutics* 15(1), 65–75. 2009. https://doi.org/10.1111/j.1755-5949.2008.00065.x

Maroon, J., & Bost, J. "Review of the Neurological Benefits of Phytocannabinoids." *Surgical neurology international* 9(91). 2018. https://doi.org/10.4103/sni.sni_45_18

MS Society of Canada. "About MS Symptoms." July 10, 2020. https://mssociety.ca/about-ms/symptoms

Peprah K, McCormack S. "Medical Cannabis for the Treatment of Dementia: A Review of Clinical Effectiveness and Guidelines." Ottawa (ON): *Canadian Agency for Drugs and Technologies in Health.* July 17, 2019. https://www.ncbi.nlm.nih.gov/books/NBK546328/

Pietrangelo, A. "Understanding Multiple Sclerosis (MS)." Healthline. May 15, 2020. https://www.healthline.com/health/multiple-sclerosis#diagnosis

"Understanding Parkinson's." Parkinson Canada. July 11, 2021. https://www.parkinson.ca/about-parkinsons/understanding-parkinsons/

Venderová K., Růzicka E., Vorísek V., Visnovský P. "Survey on Cannabis Use in Parkinson's Disease: Subjective Improvement of Motor Symptoms." Mov Disord 19(9):1102-6. September 2004. https://pubmed.ncbi.nlm.nih.gov/15372606/

SMART Goals

Devitt-Lee, A. "CBD-Drug Interactions: Role of Cytochrome P450." Retrieved July 17, 2020. https://www.projectcbd.org/medicine/cbd-drug-interactions/p450

Harvard Medical School. "CBD and Other Medications: Proceed with Caution." Retrieved September 10th, 2021. https://www.health.harvard.edu/blog/cbd-and-other-medications-proceed-with-caution-2021011121743

Iffland K, Grotenhermen F. "An Update on Safety and Side Effects of Cannabidiol: A Review of Clinical Data and Relevant Animal Studies." *Cannabis Cannabinoid Res.* 1;2(1):139-154. June 1, 2017. http://doi.org/10.1089/can.2016.0034. PMID: 28861514; PMCID: PMC5569602.

Leweke FM, Piomelli D, Pahlisch F, Muhl D, Gerth CW, Hoyer C, Klosterkötter J, Hellmich M, Koethe D. "Cannabidiol Enhances Anandamide Signaling and Alleviates Psychotic Symptoms of Schizophrenia." Transl Psychiatry. 2(3): e94. March 20, 2012. http://doi.org/10.1038/tp.2012.15. PMID: 22832859; PMCID: PMC3316151.

MindTools. "SMART Goals—How to Make Your Goals Achievable." Mindtools. Emerald Works. May 17, 2021. https://www.mindtools.com/pages/article/smart-goals.htm

Nichols, J. M., & Kaplan, B. (2020). "Immune Responses Regulated by Cannabidiol." *Cannabis and Cannabinoid Research* 5(1), 12–31. 2020. https://doi.org/10.1089/can.2018.0073

Parihar V, Rogers A, Blain AM, Zacharias SRK, Patterson LL, Siyam MA. "Reduction in Tamoxifen Metabolites Endoxifen and N-desmethyltamoxifen with Chronic Administration of Low Dose Cannabidiol: A CYP3A4 and CYP2D6 Drug Interaction." J Pharm Pract. 2020 Nov 15:897190020972208. http://doi.org/10.1177/0897190020972208.

Scherma, M., Masia, P., Satta, V. et al. "Brain Activity of Anandamide: A Rewarding Bliss?" *Acta Pharmacol Sin* 40, 309–323. 2019. https://doi.org/10.1038/s41401-018-0075-x

THC

Antoniou, Tony. "Drug interactions with Cannabinoids." *Canadian Medical Association Journal.* 192 (9) E206. March 2, 2020. Retrieved October 11, 2020. https://doi.org/10.1503/cmaj.191097

Atakan, Zerrin. "Cannabis, a Complex Plant: Different Compounds and Different Effects on Individuals." Department of Psychosis Studies, Institute of Psychiatry, King's College London. December 2, 2012. Retrieved May 10th, 2020. https://journals.sagepub.com/doi/10.1177/2045125312457586

Government of Canada. "Health Effects of Cannabis." June 5, 2020. https://www.canada.ca/content/dam/hc-sc/documents/services/campaigns/27-16-1808-Factsheet-Health-Effects-eng-web.pdf

Ryan, Sheryl A., Seth D. Ammerman, and Mary E. O'Connor. "Marijuana Use during Pregnancy and Breastfeeding: Implications for Neonatal and Childhood Outcomes." *Pediatrics* 142 (3): e20181889. 2018. https://doi.org/10.1542/peds.2018-1889.

Zou S, Kumar U. "Cannabinoid Receptors and the Endocannabinoid System: Signaling and Function in the Central Nervous System." *International Journal of Molecular Sciences.* 19(3):833. 2018. https://doi.org/10.3390/ijms19030833

Terpenes

Agus, H. H. "Terpene Toxicity and Oxidative Stress." *Toxicology*, 33–42. 2021. https://doi.org/10.1016/B978-0-12-819092-0.00004-2

Białoń, M., Krzyśko-Łupicka, T., Nowakowska-Bogdan, E., & Wieczorek, P. P. "Chemical Composition of Two Different Lavender Essential Oils and Their Effect on Facial Skin Microbiota." *Molecules* (Basel, Switzerland), 24(18), 3270. 2019. https://doi.org/10.3390/molecules24183270

Hashiesh HM, Sharma C, Goyal SN, Sadek B, Jha NK, Kaabi JA, Ojha S. "A focused Review on CB2 Receptor-Selective Pharmacological Properties and Therapeutic Potential of β-caryophyllene, a Dietary Cannabinoid." *Biomed Pharmacother.* 2021 Aug;140:111639. http://doi.org/10.1016/j.biopha.2021.111639

Khaleel, C., Tabanca, N. & Buchbauer, G. "α-Terpineol, a Natural Monoterpene: a Review of Its Biological Properties." *Open Chemistry* 16(1), 349-361. 2018. https://doi.org/10.1515/chem-2018-0040

Lillehei A.S., Halcón, L.L. "A Systematic Review of the Effect of Inhaled Essential Oils on Sleep." *J Altern Complement Med* 20(6):441-51. June 2014. http://doi.org/10.1089/acm.2013.0311

Lillehei, A. S., Halcón, L. L., Savik, K., & Reis, R. "Effect of Inhaled Lavender and Sleep Hygiene on Self-Reported Sleep Issues: a Randomized Controlled Trial." *Journal of Alternative and Complementary Medicine* (New York, N.Y.), 21(7), 430–438. 2015. https://doi.org/10.1089/acm.2014.0327

Rogerio AP, Andrade EL, Leite DF, Figueiredo CP, Calixto JB. "Preventive and Therapeutic Anti-Inflammatory Properties of the Sesquiterpene Alpha-Humulene in Experimental Airways Allergic Inflammation." *Br J Pharmacol.* 158(4):1074-87. October 2009. http://doi.org/10.1111/j.1476-5381.2009.00177.x

Russo, E. B. "Taming THC: Potential Cannabis Synergy and Phytocannabinoid-Terpenoid Entourage Effects." *British Journal of Pharmacology* 163(7), 1344–1364. 2011. https://doi.org/10.1111/j.1476-5381.2011.01238.x

Sobel, Ashley. "What is Limonene? Everything You Need to Know." Healthline. Retrieved July 17, 2020. https://www.healthline.com/nutrition/d-limonene

Weston-Green, K., Class, H. and Naranjo, C.J. "A Review of the Potential Use of Pinene and Linalool as Terpene-Based Medicines for Brain Health: Discovering Novel Therapeutics in the Flavours and Fragrances of Cannabis." *Frontiers in Psychiatry* 12(August). August 26, 2021. https://doi.org/10.3389/fpsyt.2021.583211

Wellness

Global Wellness Institute. "What is Wellness?" Retrieved November 14, 2021. https://globalwellnessinstitute.org/what-is-wellness/

Institute for Work & Health. "Primary, Secondary and Tertiary Prevention." April 2015. Retrieved July 7, 2021. https://www.iwh.on.ca/what-researchers-mean-by/primary-secondary-and-tertiary-prevention

World Health Organization. "Social Determinants of Health." Retrieved August 12, 2021. https://www.who.int/health-topics/social-determinants-of-health#tab=tab_1

World Health Organization (1948). "WHO Definition of Health: Preamble to the Constitution of the World Health Organization." Retrieved May 15, 2021. https://www.who.int/governance/eb/who_constitution_en.pdf

CPSIA information can be obtained
at www.ICGtesting.com
Printed in the USA
LVHW080326160422
716314LV00018B/835/J

9 780228 840916